Neurology Residency Match Selection Criteria
and Programs Requirements

By

Match A Doc
and
Residency Guide

Table of Contents

Introduction 15

Alabama 19

    University of South Alabama Neurology Residency Program 19

    University of Alabama Medical Center Neurology Residency Program..................20

Arizona 21

    University of Arizona College of Medicine at South Campus Neurology Residency Program 21

    University of Arizona Neurology Residency Program..22

    St Joseph's Hospital and Medical Center Neurology Residency Program..................23

Mayo Clinic College of Medicine (Arizona) Neurology Residency Program......................24

Arkansas...25

University of Arkansas for Medical Sciences Neurology Residency Program......................25

California..26

Cedars-Sinai Medical Center Neurology Residency Program 26

Loma Linda University Neurology Residency Program..27

Stanford University Neurology Residency Program..28

University of California (San Francisco) Neurology Residency Program......................29

University of California (San Diego) Neurology Residency Program 30

UCLA Medical Center Neurology Residency Program..31

University of Southern California/LAC+USC Medical Center Neurology Residency Program..32

University of California (Irvine) Neurology Residency Program 33

Kaiser Permanente Southern California (Los Angeles) Neurology Residency Program......34

University of California (Davis) Health System Neurology Residency Program.....................35

Los Angeles County-Harbor-UCLA Medical Center Neurology Residency Program.........36

Colorado...37

University of Colorado Neurology Residency Program...37

Connecticut..38

University of Connecticut Neurology Residency Program 38

Yale-New Haven Medical Center Neurology Residency Program 39

District of Columbia 40

Howard University Neurology Residency Program...40

George Washington University Neurology Residency Program 41

Georgetown University Hospital Neurology Residency Program 42

Florida 43

Cleveland Clinic (Florida) Neurology
Residency Program 43

University of South Florida Morsani
Neurology Residency Program.....................44

Jackson Memorial Hospital/Jackson Health
System Neurology Residency Program 45

University of Florida Neurology Residency
Program...46

Mayo Clinic College of Medicine (Jacksonville)
Neurology Residency Program.....................47

University of Florida College of Medicine
Jacksonville Neurology Residency Program.48

Georgia..49

Medical College of Georgia Neurology
Residency Program 49

Emory University Neurology Residency
Program...50

Illinois..51

University of Illinois College of Medicine at
Peoria Neurology Residency Program 51

Southern Illinois University Neurology
Residency Program 52

Loyola University Neurology Residency
Program...53

University of Illinois College of Medicine at Chicago Neurology Residency Program 54

University of Chicago Neurology Residency Neurology Program 55

McGaw Medical Center of Northwestern University Neurology Residency Program ... 56

Rush University Medical Center Neurology Residency Program 57

Indiana 58

Indiana University School of Medicine Neurology Residency Program 58

Iowa 59

University of Iowa Hospitals and Clinics Neurology Residency Program 59

Kansas 60

University of Kansas School of Medicine Neurology Residency Program 61

Kentucky 62

University of Louisville Neurology Residency Program 62

University of Kentucky College of Medicine Neurology Residency Program 63

Louisiana 64

Louisiana State University (Shreveport) Neurology Residency Program......................64

Tulane University Neurology Residency Program...65

Louisiana State University Neurology Residency Program 66

Ochsner Clinic Foundation Neurology Residency Program 67

Maryland...68

University of Maryland Neurology Residency Program...68

Johns Hopkins University Neurology Residency Program 69

Massachusetts 70

Massachusetts General Hospital/Brigham and Women's Hospital/Harvard Medical School Neurology Residency Program......................70

Boston Medical Center Neurology Residency Program...71

University of Massachusetts Neurology Residency Program 72

Tufts Medical Center Neurology Residency Program...73

Beth Israel Deaconess Medical Center/Harvard Medical School Neurology Residency Program 74

Michigan...75

Detroit Medical Center/Wayne State University Neurology Residency Program ...75

University of Michigan Neurology Residency Program..76

Sparrow Hospital/Michigan State University Neurology Residency Program......................77

Henry Ford Hospital/Wayne State University Neurology Residency Program......................78

Grand Rapids Medical Education Partners Neurology Residency Program......................79

Minnesota 80

Mayo Clinic College of Medicine (Rochester) Neurology Residency Program......................80

University of Minnesota Neurology Residency Program..81

Mississippi...82

University of Mississippi Medical Center Neurology Residency Program......................82

Missouri 83

Washington University/B-JH/SLCH Consortium Neurology Residency Program.83

St Louis University School of Medicine Neurology Residency Program......................84

University of Missouri-Columbia Neurology Residency Program 85

Nebraska 86

University of Nebraska Medical Center College of Medicine/Creighton University Neurology Residency Program......................86

New Hampshire...87

Dartmouth-Hitchcock Medical Center Neurology Residency Program......................87

New Jersey 88

Cooper Medical School of Rowan University/Cooper University Hospital Neurology Residency Program......................88

Rutgers New Jersey Medical School Neurology Residency Program......................89

Seton Hall University School of Health and Medical Sciences Neurology Residency Program...90

Rutgers Robert Wood Johnson Medical School Neurology Residency Program 91

New Mexico 92

  University of New Mexico Neurology
Residency Program 92

New York 94

  Icahn School of Medicine at Mount Sinai
(Beth Israel) Neurology Residency Program 94

  Albany Medical Center Neurology Residency
Program 95

  University at Buffalo Neurology Residency
Program 96

  Albert Einstein College of Medicine
Neurology Residency Program 97

  New York Presbyterian Hospital (Cornell
Campus) Neurology Residency Program 98

  NSLIJHS/Hofstra North Shore-LIJ School of
Medicine Neurology Residency Program 99

  Icahn School of Medicine at Mount Sinai
Neurology Residency Program 100

  New York Medical College at Westchester
Medical Center Neurology Program 101

  New York University School of Medicine
Neurology Residency Program 102

  SUNY Health Science Center at Brooklyn
Neurology Residency Program 103

SUNY at Stony Brook Neurology Residency Program...104

SUNY Upstate Medical University Neurology Residency Program 105

New York Presbyterian Hospital (Columbia Campus) Neurology Residency Program....106

University of Rochester Neurology Residency Program...107

North Carolina..108

Wake Forest University School of Medicine Neurology Residency Program....................108

Duke University Hospital Neurology Residency Program 109

University of North Carolina Hospitals Neurology Residency Program....................110

Ohio...111

Wright State University Boonshoft School of Medicine Neurology Residency Program...111

Cleveland Clinic Foundation Neurology Residency Program 112

University of Cincinnati Medical Center/College of Medicine Neurology Rresidency Program 113

Case Western Reserve University/University Hospitals Case Medical Center Neurology Residency Program 114

Ohio State University Hospital Neurology Residency Program 115

University of Toledo Neurology Residency Program..116

Oklahoma..117

University of Oklahoma Health Sciences Center Neurology Residency Program.......117

Oregon 118

Oregon Health & Science University Neurology Residency Program...................118

Pennsylvania 119

Geisinger Health System Neurology Residency Program 119

Penn State Milton S Hershey Medical Center Neurology Residency Program...................120

Drexel University College of Medicine/Hahnemann University Hospital Neurology Residency Program...................121

Temple University Hospital Neurology Residency Program 122

Thomas Jefferson University Neurology Residency Program 123

University of Pennsylvania Neurology Residency Program 124

UPMC Medical Education Neurology Residency Program 125

Allegheny General Hospital-Western Pennsylvania Hospital Medical Education Consortium (AGH) Neurology Residency Program 126

Albert Einstein Healthcare Network Neurology Residency Program 127

Rhode Island 128

Brown University Neurology Residency Program 128

South Carolina 129

Palmetto Health/University of South Carolina School of Medicine Neurology Residency Program 129

Medical University of South Carolina Neurology Residency Program 130

Tennessee 131

University of Tennessee Neurology Residency Program 131

Vanderbilt University Neurology Residency Program 132

Texas 133

Scott and White Memorial Hospital Neurology Residency Program 134

University of Texas Medical Branch Hospitals Neurology Residency Program 134

University of Texas Southwestern Medical School (Austin) Neurology Residency Program 135

Methodist Hospital (Houston) Neurology Residency Program 136

Texas Tech University (Lubbock) Neurology Residency Program 137

University of Texas Southwestern Medical School Neurology Residency Program 138

Baylor College of Medicine Neurology Residency Program 139

University of Texas Health Science Center at San Antonio Neurology Residency Program 140

University of Texas at Houston Neurology Residency Program 141

Utah 142

University of Utah Neurology Residency Program 142

Vermont 143

University of Vermont/Fletcher Allen Health Care Neurology Residency Program 143

Virginia 144

Virginia Commonwealth University Health System Neurology Residency Program 144

University of Virginia Neurology Residency Program 145

Washington 146

University of Washington Neurology Residency Program 146

West Virginia 148

West Virginia University Neurology Residency Program 148

Wisconsin 149

Medical College of Wisconsin Affiliated Hospitals Neurology Residency Program ... 149

University of Wisconsin Neurology Residency Program 150

Introduction

Neurology Residency Match Selection Criteria and Programs Requirements

This book is the must-read book and most single important piece you buy in your battle for residency. This is the **Neurology** Residency Match Selection Criteria and

Programs Requirements book that contains up-to-date information about all the programs in the United States for both AMGs and IMGs. Why this book is essential to match? It has been shown that applying to programs that you don't match their minimum criteria is just waste of money and time. It is very important that you apply to those programs that you meet their requirements and this why we decided to make your life easier by gathering the information you need in one book. The information was gathered from program directors, coordinators, chiefs, faculty and residents. It includes Programs names, Programs codes, States, Addresses, Phones, Faxes, Percentage of IMGs in the programs, Minimum USMLE Step 1 and Step 2 Score Requirements, Attempts on any step, CS requirement at time of application, USCE

Requirements, Cut-Off time since graduation, Programs offering couple match and Visas Sponsored or accepted. We have more than 10 years experience in the match field and our book is the proof that will help you to get the highest number of interviews to increase your chances in the match journey.

Disclaimer: We are not affiliated to any official or non official organization. We are not affiliated to ECFMG, ERAS, NRMP or USMLE.

Disclaimer: The information in this book is personally collected by the author from various resources in the residency programs which is/are subject to change by/at the programs at any time. Although we did our best to get the most accurate information as much as possible from the program directors, coordinators, faculty and residents, however, you understand that by reading this book you are using the information here on your own responsibility.

Alabama

University of South Alabama Neurology Residency Program

Specialty: Neurology
Program name: University of South Alabama Program
Program code: 180-01-21-123
Program type: University-based
State: Alabama
Address: University of South Alabama Medical Center,
   Department of Neurology 10th Floor Suite E,
   2451 Fillingim St, Mobile, AL 36617
Phone: (251) 445-8261
Fax: (251) 445-8249
Percentage of IMGs in the program: 35%
Minimum USMLE Step 1 Score Requirement: 206
Minimum USMLE Step 2 Score Requirement: 206
Attempts on any step: No limits set
CS required at time of application: No
USCE Requirement: No
Cut-Off time since graduation: 5 years
Program offers couple match: Yes
Visas Sponsored or accepted: J1 visa

University of Alabama Medical Center Neurology Residency Program

Specialty: Neurology
Program name: University of Alabama Medical Center Program
Program code: 180-01-31-004
NRMP Code: 1007180C0
Program type: University-based
State: Alabama
Address: University of Alabama Medical Center, Sparks Ctr 440,
 1720 7th Ave S, Birmingham, AL 35294-0017
Phone: (205) 975-0447
Fax: (205) 996-4150
Percentage of IMGs in the program: 30%
Minimum USMLE Step 1 Score Requirement: 204
Minimum USMLE Step 2 Score Requirement: 204
Attempts on any step: Must pass on first attempt including CS exam
CS required at time of application: Yes
USCE Requirement: None
Cut-Off time since graduation: 5 years
Program offers couple match: Yes
Visas Sponsored or accepted: J1 visa and H1b visa

Arizona

University of Arizona College of Medicine at South Campus Neurology Residency Program

Specialty: Neurology
Program name: University of Arizona College of Medicine at South Campus Program
Program code: 180-03-31-159
NRMP Code: 1371180C0
Program type: University-based
State: Arizona
Address: University of Arizona Medical Center South Campus
 2800 E Ajo Way, Tucson, AZ 85713
Phone: (520) 874-4217
Fax: (520) 874-4226
Percentage of IMGs in the program: 50%
Minimum USMLE Step 1 Score Requirement: 215
Minimum USMLE Step 2 Score Requirement: 215
Attempts on any step: No limits set
CS required at time of application: Yes
USCE Requirement: None
Cut-Off time since graduation: 10 years

Program offers couple match: Yes
Visas Sponsored or accepted: J1 visa

University of Arizona Neurology Residency Program

Specialty: Neurology
Program name: University of Arizona Program
Program code: 180-03-21-006
NRMP Code: 1015180C0
Program type: University-based
State: Arizona
Address: University of Arizona College of Medicine
 1501 N Campbell Ave, Tucson, AZ 85724-5023
Phone: (520) 626-3894
Fax: (520) 626-2111
Percentage of IMGs in the program: 40%
Minimum USMLE Step 1 Score Requirement: No limits set
Minimum USMLE Step 2 Score Requirement: No limits set
Attempts on any step: No limits set
CS required at time of application: Yes
USCE Requirement: None
Cut-Off time since graduation: 5 years
Program offers couple match: Yes
Visas Sponsored or accepted: J1 visa

St Joseph's Hospital and Medical Center Neurology Residency Program

Specialty: Neurology
Program name: St Joseph's Hospital and Medical Center Program
Program code: 180-03-12-005
NRMP Code: 1012180A0
Program type: Community-based University affiliated hospital
State: Arizona
Address: St Joseph's Hospital and Medical Center
350 W Thomas Rd, Phoenix, AZ 85013
Phone: (602) 406-3450
Fax: (602) 798-0467
Percentage of IMGs in the program: 10%
Minimum USMLE Step 1 Score Requirement: No limits set
Minimum USMLE Step 2 Score Requirement: No limits set
Attempts on any step: No limits set
CS required at time of application: No
USCE Requirement: None
Cut-Off time since graduation: 10 years
Program offers couple match: Yes
Visas Sponsored or accepted: J1 visa

Mayo Clinic College of Medicine (Arizona) Neurology Residency Program

Specialty: Neurology
Program name: Mayo Clinic College of Medicine (Arizona) Program
Program code: 180-03-11-150
NRMP Code: 3200180C0
Program type: Community-based University affiliated hospital
State: Arizona
Address: Mayo Clinic Arizona
   13400 E Shea Blvd, Scottsdale, AZ 85259
Phone: (480) 301-4395
Fax: (480) 301-9776
Percentage of IMGs in the program: 0%
Minimum USMLE Step 1 Score Requirement: 225
Minimum USMLE Step 2 Score Requirement: 225
Attempts on any step: No limits set
CS required at time of application: No
USCE Requirement: None
Cut-Off time since graduation: 5 years
Program offers couple match: Yes
Visas Sponsored or accepted: J1 visa and H1b visa

Arkansas

University of Arkansas for Medical Sciences Neurology Residency Program

Specialty: Neurology
Program name: University of Arkansas for Medical Sciences Program
Program code: 180-04-21-007
State: Arkansas
Address: University of Arkansas for Medical Sciences
    4301 W Markham St, Little Rock, AR 72205
Phone: (501) 686-5135
Fax: (501) 686-8689
Percentage of IMGs in the program: 40%
Minimum USMLE Step 1 Score Requirement: No limits set
Minimum USMLE Step 2 Score Requirement: No limits set
Attempts on any step: No limits set
CS required at time of application: Yes including ECFMG certificate
USCE Requirement: None

Cut-Off time since graduation: 8 years
Program offers couple match: Yes
Visas Sponsored or accepted: J1 visa

California

Cedars-Sinai Medical Center Neurology Residency Program

Specialty: Neurology
Program name: Cedars-Sinai Medical Center Program
Program code: 180-05-21-165
State: California
Address: Cedars-Sinai Medical Center
127 S San Vicente Blvd, Los Angeles, CA 90048
Phone: (310) 248-6842
Fax: (310) 967-0601
Percentage of IMGs in the program: 30%
Minimum USMLE Step 1 Score Requirement: No limits set
Minimum USMLE Step 2 Score Requirement: No limits set

Attempts on any step: No limits set
CS required at time of application: Yes including ECFMG certificate and PTAL/Status letter
USCE Requirement: None
Cut-Off time since graduation: No limits set
Program offers couple match: Yes
Visas Sponsored or accepted: J1 visa

Loma Linda University Neurology Residency Program

Specialty: Neurology
Program name: Loma Linda University Program
Program code: 180-05-21-124
State: California
Address: Loma Linda University Medical Center 11175 Campus St, Loma Linda, CA 92354
Phone: (909) 558-4907
Fax: (909) 558-0207
Percentage of IMGs in the program: 50%
Minimum USMLE Step 1 Score Requirement: 210 (190 previously)
Minimum USMLE Step 2 Score Requirement: 210 (190 previously)
Attempts on any step: Must pass on maximum 2nd attempt including CS exam

CS required at time of application: Yes including ECFMG certificate and PTAL/Status letter
USCE Requirement: None
Cut-Off time since graduation: 10 years but must be clinically active
Program offers couple match: Yes
Visas Sponsored or accepted: J1 visa

Stanford University Neurology Residency Program

Specialty: Neurology
Program name: Stanford University Program
Program code: 180-05-21-017
NRMP Code: 1820180A0
Program type: University-based
State: California
Address: Stanford University Medical Center
300 Pasteur Dr, Stanford, CA 94305-5235
Phone: (650) 725-6688
Fax: (650) 725-7459
Percentage of IMGs in the program: 0%.
Minimum USMLE Step 1 Score Requirement: No limits set
Minimum USMLE Step 2 Score Requirement: No limits set
Attempts on any step: No limits set

CS required at time of application: Yes including ECFMG certificate and PTAL/Status letter. IMGs must be done with Step 3 before applying.
USCE Requirement: Yes, 6 months
Cut-Off time since graduation: No limits set
Program offers couple match: No
Visas Sponsored or accepted: J1 visa

University of California (San Francisco) Neurology Residency Program

Specialty: Neurology
Program name: University of California (San Francisco) Program
Program code: 180-05-21-016
State: California
Address: UCSF Medical Center
505 Parnassus Ave, San Francisco, CA 94143-0114
Phone: (415) 476-3891
Fax: (415) 476-3428
Percentage of IMGs in the program: 0%
Minimum USMLE Step 1 Score Requirement: No limits set
Minimum USMLE Step 2 Score Requirement: No limits set
Attempts on any step: Must pass on first attempt

CS required at time of application: No but PTAL/Status letter is required
USCE Requirement: Yes, 2 months
Cut-Off time since graduation: 5 years
Program offers couple match: Yes
Visas Sponsored or accepted: J1 visa

University of California (San Diego) Neurology Residency Program

Specialty: Neurology
Program name: University of California (San Diego) Program
Program code: 180-05-21-014
NRMP Code: 1049180A0
Program type: University-based
State: California
Address: UCSD Medical Center
200 W Arbor Dr, San Diego, CA 92103-8465
Phone: (619) 543-6266
Fax: (619) 543-5793
Percentage of IMGs in the program: 20%
Minimum USMLE Step 1 Score Requirement: 235
Minimum USMLE Step 2 Score Requirement: 235
Attempts on any step: Must pass on first attempt

CS required at time of application: Yes including ECFMG certificate and PTAL/Status letter
USCE Requirement: None
Cut-Off time since graduation: No limits set
Program offers couple match: Yes
Visas Sponsored or accepted: J1 visa

UCLA Medical Center Neurology Residency Program

Specialty: Neurology
Program name: UCLA Medical Center Program
Program code: 180-05-21-012
State: California
Address: UCLA Medical Center
710 Westwood Plaza, Los Angeles, CA 90025
Phone: (310) 825-0703
Fax: (310) 206-4733
Percentage of IMGs in the program: 0%
Minimum USMLE Step 1 Score Requirement: No limits set
Minimum USMLE Step 2 Score Requirement: No limits set
Attempts on any step: No limits set
CS required at time of application: Yes including ECFMG certificate and PTAL/Status letter

USCE Requirement: None
Cut-Off time since graduation: No limits set
Program offers couple match: Yes
Visas Sponsored or accepted: J1 visa

University of Southern California/LAC+USC Medical Center Neurology Residency Program

Specialty: Neurology
Program name: University of Southern California/LAC+USC Medical Center Program
Program code: 180-05-21-011
NRMP Code: 1033180A0
Program type: University-based
State: California
Address: LAC+USC Medical Center
1200 N State St, Los Angeles, CA 90033
Phone: (323) 409-4535
Fax: (323) 441-8093
Percentage of IMGs in the program: 10%
Minimum USMLE Step 1 Score Requirement: No limits set
Minimum USMLE Step 2 Score Requirement: No limits set
Attempts on any step: No limits set

CS required at time of application: Yes including ECFMG certificate and PTAL/Status letter
USCE Requirement: None
Cut-Off time since graduation: No limits set
Program offers couple match: Yes
Visas Sponsored or accepted: J1 visa

University of California (Irvine) Neurology Residency Program

Specialty: Neurology
Program name: University of California (Irvine) Program
Program code: 180-05-21-009
NRMP Code: 1043180A0
Program type: University-based
State: California
Address: UC Irvine Medical Center
200 S Manchester Ave, Orange, CA 92868
Phone: (714) 456-7707
Fax: (714) 456-8805
Percentage of IMGs in the program: 20%
Minimum USMLE Step 1 Score Requirement: No limits set
Minimum USMLE Step 2 Score Requirement: No limits set

Attempts on any step: Must pass on first attempt
CS required at time of application: Yes including ECFMG certificate and PTAL/Status letter
USCE Requirement: None
Cut-Off time since graduation: No limits set
Program offers couple match: Yes
Visas Sponsored or accepted: No visa

Kaiser Permanente Southern California (Los Angeles) Neurology Residency Program

Specialty: Neurology
Program name: Kaiser Permanente Southern California (Los Angeles) Program
Program code: 180-05-12-010
State: California
Address: Kaiser Permanente Medical Care
393 E Walnut St, Pasadena, CA 91188
Phone: (323) 783-8883
Fax: (626) 405-6581
Percentage of IMGs in the program: 10%
Minimum USMLE Step 1 Score Requirement: No limits set
Minimum USMLE Step 2 Score Requirement: No limits set
Attempts on any step: No limits set

CS required at time of application: Yes including ECFMG certificate and PTAL/Status letter
USCE Requirement: None
Cut-Off time since graduation: No limits set
Program offers couple match: Yes
Visas Sponsored or accepted: No visa

University of California (Davis) Health System Neurology Residency Program

Specialty: Neurology
Program name: University of California (Davis) Health System Program
Program code: 180-05-12-008
Program type: University-based
State: California
Address: UC Davis Medical Centre
 4860 Y St, Sacramento, CA 95817
Phone: (916) 734-3514
Fax: (916) 734-6525
Percentage of IMGs in the program: 10%
Minimum USMLE Step 1 Score Requirement: No limits set
Minimum USMLE Step 2 Score Requirement: No limits set
Attempts on any step: Must pass on first attempt

CS required at time of application: No but PTAL/Status letter required
USCE Requirement: None
Cut-Off time since graduation: 5 years
Program offers couple match: Yes
Visas Sponsored or accepted: J1 visa

Los Angeles County-Harbor-UCLA Medical Center Neurology Residency Program

Specialty: Neurology
Program name: Los Angeles County-UCLA Medical Center Program
Program code: 180-05-11-018
NRMP Code: 1067180A0
Program type: University-based
State: California
Address: Los Angeles County-Harbor-UCLA Medical Center
1000 W Carson St, Torrance, CA 90509
Phone: (310) 222-3897
Fax: (310) 533-8905
Percentage of IMGs in the program: 10%
Minimum USMLE Step 1 Score Requirement: No limits set
Minimum USMLE Step 2 Score Requirement: No limits set
Attempts on any step: No limit set

CS required at time of application: Yes including ECFMG certificate and PTAL/Status letter
USCE Requirement: Yes, 8 months
Cut-Off time since graduation: No limits set
Program offers couple match: Yes
Visas Sponsored or accepted: J1 visa

Colorado

University of Colorado Neurology Residency Program

Specialty: Neurology
Program name: University of Colorado Program
Program code: 180-07-21-019
State: Colorado
Address: University of Colorado Denver School of Medicine
    12700 E 19th Ave, Aurora, CO 80045
Phone: (303) 724-4330
Fax: (303) 724-4764
Percentage of IMGs in the program: 0% (occasionally one)
Minimum USMLE Step 1 Score Requirement: No limits set

Minimum USMLE Step 2 Score Requirement: No limits set
Attempts on any step: Must pass on first attempt
CS required at time of application: Yes including ECFMG certificate
USCE Requirement: None
Cut-Off time since graduation: 5 years
Program offers couple match: Yes
Visas Sponsored or accepted: J1 visa

Connecticut

University of Connecticut Neurology Residency Program

Specialty: Neurology
Program name: University of Connecticut Program
Program code: 180-08-21-139
NRMP Code: 1094180C0
Program type: Community-based university affiliated hospital
State: Connecticut

Address: Hartford Hospital
80 Seymour St, Hartford, CT 06102-5037
Phone: (860) 545-5120
Fax: (860) 545-5003
Percentage of IMGs in the program: 90%
Minimum USMLE Step 1 Score Requirement: 210
Minimum USMLE Step 2 Score Requirement: 210
Attempts on any step: Must pass on first attempt
CS required at time of application: No
USCE Requirement: None
Cut-Off time since graduation: 5 years
Program offers couple match: Yes
Visas Sponsored or accepted: J1 visa

Yale-New Haven Medical Center Neurology Residency Program

Specialty: Neurology
Program name: Yale-New Haven Medical Center Program
Program code: 180-08-21-021
NRMP Code: 1089180A0, 1089180A1
Program type: University-based
State: Connecticut
Address: Yale-New Haven Medical Center
15 York St, New Haven, CT 06520

Phone: (203) 785-6054
Fax: (203) 785-6246
Percentage of IMGs in the program: 10%
Minimum USMLE Step 1 Score Requirement: 215
Minimum USMLE Step 2 Score Requirement: 210
Attempts on any step: No limits set
CS required at time of application: No
USCE Requirement: None
Cut-Off time since graduation: 5 years
Program offers couple match: Yes
Visas Sponsored or accepted: J1 visa and H1b visa

District of Columbia

Howard University Neurology Residency Program

Specialty: Neurology
Program name: Howard University Program
Program code: 180-10-21-024
State: District of Columbia
Address: Howard University Hospital
2041 Georgia Ave NW, Washington,

DC 20060
Phone: (202) 865-1546
Fax: (202) 865-4395
Percentage of IMGs in the program: 50%
Minimum USMLE Step 1 Score Requirement: No limits set
Minimum USMLE Step 2 Score Requirement: No limits set
Attempts on any step: Must pass maximum on 2nd attempt including CS exam
CS required at time of application: Yes including ECFMG certificate
USCE Requirement: None
Cut-Off time since graduation: No limits set
Program offers couple match: No
Visas Sponsored or accepted: J1 visa and H1b visa

George Washington University Neurology Residency Program

Specialty: Neurology
Program name: George Washington University Program
Program code: 180-10-21-023
State: District of Columbia
Address: George Washington University Medical Center
          2150 Pennsylvania Ave NW, Washington, DC 20037

Phone: (202) 741-3411
Fax: (202) 741-2721
Percentage of IMGs in the program: 50%
Minimum USMLE Step 1 Score Requirement: No limits set
Minimum USMLE Step 2 Score Requirement: No limits set
Attempts on any step: No limits set
CS required at time of application: Yes including ECFMG certificate
USCE Requirement: Yes
Cut-Off time since graduation: No limits set
Program offers couple match: Yes
Visas Sponsored or accepted: J1 visa

Georgetown University Hospital Neurology Residency Program

Specialty: Neurology
Program name: Georgetown University Hospital Program
Program code: 180-10-21-022
State: District of Columbia
Address: Georgetown University Hospital
3800 Reservoir Rd NW, Washington, DC 20007
Phone: (202) 444-1037
Fax: (202) 444-2813
Percentage of IMGs in the program: 10%

Minimum USMLE Step 1 Score Requirement:
No limits set
Minimum USMLE Step 2 Score Requirement:
No limits set
Attempts on any step: No limits set
CS required at time of application: No
USCE Requirement: Yes
Cut-Off time since graduation: No limits set
Program offers couple match: Yes
Visas Sponsored or accepted: J1 visa

Florida

Cleveland Clinic (Florida) Neurology Residency Program

Specialty: Neurology
Program name: Cleveland Clinic (Florida) Program
Program code: 180-11-22-152
NRMP Code: 1383180A0
Program type: Community-based
State: Florida
Address: Cleveland Clinic Florida
2950 Cleveland Clinic Blvd, Weston, FL 33331

Phone: (954) 659-5359
Fax: (954) 659-6216
Percentage of IMGs in the program: 80%
Minimum USMLE Step 1 Score Requirement: 210
Minimum USMLE Step 2 Score Requirement: 210
Attempts on any step: Must pass on first attempt
CS required at time of application: Yes including ECFMG certificate
USCE Requirement: Yes
Cut-Off time since graduation: No limits set
Program offers couple match: No
Visas Sponsored or accepted: J1 visa and H1b visa

University of South Florida Morsani Neurology Residency Program

Specialty: Neurology
Program name: University of South Florida Morsani Program
Program code: 180-11-21-027
NRMP Code: 1109180C0
Program type: Community-based university affiliated hospital
State: Florida
Address: James A Haley Veterans Hospital
13000 Bruce B Downs Blvd, Tampa, FL

33612-4798
Phone: (813) 972-2000   Ext: 7085
Fax: (813) 978-5995
Percentage of IMGs in the program: 25%
Minimum USMLE Step 1 Score Requirement: 225
Minimum USMLE Step 2 Score Requirement: 225
Attempts on any step: No limits set
CS required at time of application: Yes including ECFMG certificate
USCE Requirement: None
Cut-Off time since graduation: 5 years
Program offers couple match: Yes
Visas Sponsored or accepted: J1 visa

Jackson Memorial Hospital/Jackson Health System Neurology Residency Program

Specialty: Neurology
Program name: Jackson Memorial Hospital/Jackson Health System Program
Program code: 180-11-21-026
State: Florida
Address: Jackson Memorial Hospital
            1120 NW 14th St, Miami, FL 33136
Phone: (305) 243-2742
Fax: (305) 243-2742
Percentage of IMGs in the program: 30%

Minimum USMLE Step 1 Score Requirement: No limits set
Minimum USMLE Step 2 Score Requirement: No limits set
Attempts on any step: Must pass on first attempt including CS exam
CS required at time of application: No
USCE Requirement: None
Cut-Off time since graduation: No limits set
Program offers couple match: Yes
Visas Sponsored or accepted: J1 visa

University of Florida Neurology Residency Program

Specialty: Neurology
Program name: University of Florida Program
Program code: 180-11-21-025
State: Florida
Address: University of Florida College of Medicine
　　　　100 S Newell Dr, Gainesville, FL 32610
Phone: (352) 273-5550
Fax: (352) 273-5575
Percentage of IMGs in the program: 60%
Minimum USMLE Step 1 Score Requirement: No limits set
Minimum USMLE Step 2 Score Requirement: No limits set

Attempts on any step: Must pass on first attempt including CS exam
CS required at time of application: Yes
USCE Requirement: Yes
Cut-Off time since graduation: No limits set
Program offers couple match: Yes
Visas Sponsored or accepted: J1 visa (H1b visa for advanced positions might be considered in special situations if approved by their GME council)

Mayo Clinic College of Medicine (Jacksonville) Neurology Residency Program

Specialty: Neurology
Program name: Mayo Clinic College of Medicine (Jacksonville) Program
Program code: 180-11-13-148
NRMP Code: 1032180C0
Program type: Community-based University affiliated hospital
State: Florida
Address: Mayo Clinic Jacksonville
4500 San Pablo Rd, Jacksonville, FL 32224
Phone: (904) 953-0435
Fax: (904) 953-0430
Percentage of IMGs in the program: 0%

Minimum USMLE Step 1 Score Requirement: No limits set
Minimum USMLE Step 2 Score Requirement: No limits set
Attempts on any step: Must pass on first attempt including CS exam
CS required at time of application: No
USCE Requirement: Yes, 2 years
Cut-Off time since graduation: No limits set
Program offers couple match: Yes
Visas Sponsored or accepted: J1 visa

University of Florida College of Medicine Jacksonville Neurology Residency Program

Specialty: Neurology
Program name: University of Florida College of Medicine Jacksonville Program
Program code: 180-11-12-154
NRMP Code: 1101180A0
Program type: Community-based University affiliated hospital
State: Florida
Address: University of Florida College of Med Jacksonville
    580 W 8th St, Jacksonville, FL 32209
Phone: (904) 244-9696

Fax: (904) 244-9481
Percentage of IMGs in the program: 55%
Minimum USMLE Step 1 Score Requirement: No limits set
Minimum USMLE Step 2 Score Requirement: No limits set
Attempts on any step: No limits set
CS required at time of application: Yes including ECFMG certificate
USCE Requirement: None
Cut-Off time since graduation: No limits set
Program offers couple match: Yes
Visas Sponsored or accepted: J1 visa

Georgia

Medical College of Georgia Neurology Residency Program

Specialty: Neurology
Program name: Medical College of Georgia Program
Program code: 180-12-21-029
NRMP Code: 1985180A0
Program type: University-based
State: Georgia

Address: Georgia Regents University MCG
1120 15th St, Augusta, GA 30912-3260
Phone: (706) 721-1990
Fax: (706) 721-1221
Percentage of IMGs in the program: 50%
Minimum USMLE Step 1 Score Requirement: 220
Minimum USMLE Step 2 Score Requirement: 220
Attempts on any step: Must pass on first attempt
CS required at time of application: No
USCE Requirement: Yes, 6 months
Cut-Off time since graduation: 5 years
Program offers couple match: Yes
Visas Sponsored or accepted: J1 visa

Emory University Neurology Residency Program

Specialty: Neurology
Program name: Emory University Program
Program code: 180-12-21-028
State: Georgia
Address: Emory University Hospital
101 Woodruff Circle, Atlanta, GA 30322
Phone: (404) 727-5004

Fax: (404) 727-3157
Percentage of IMGs in the program: 15%
Minimum USMLE Step 1 Score Requirement: No limits set
Minimum USMLE Step 2 Score Requirement: No limits set
Attempts on any step: No limits set
CS required at time of application: Yes as well as ECFMG certificate
USCE Requirement: Yes
Cut-Off time since graduation: 5 years
Program offers couple match: Yes
Visas Sponsored or accepted: J1 visa and H1b visa

Illinois

University of Illinois College of Medicine at Peoria Neurology Residency Program

Specialty: Neurology
Program name: University of Illinois College of Medicine at Peoria Program
Program code: 180-16-21-147

NRMP Code: 1175180C0
Program type: Community-based university affiliated hospital
State: Illinois
Address: OSF St Francis Medical Center
530 NE Glen Oak Ave, Peoria, IL 61637
Phone: (309) 655-2702
Fax: (309) 655-3069
Percentage of IMGs in the program: 100%
Minimum USMLE Step 1 Score Requirement: No limits set
Minimum USMLE Step 2 Score Requirement: No limits set
Attempts on any step: Combined total of 5 maximum attempts together.
CS required at time of application: No
USCE Requirement: None
Cut-Off time since graduation: 5 years
Program offers couple match: Yes
Visas Sponsored or accepted: J1 visa and H1b visa

Southern Illinois University Neurology Residency Program

Specialty: Neurology
Program name: Southern Illinois University Program
Program code: 180-16-21-134

NRMP Code: 2922180C0
Program type: Community-based university affiliated hospital
State: Illinois
Address: Southern Illinois University School of Medicine
751 N Rutledge St, Springfield, IL 62794-9643
Phone: (217) 545-7210
Fax: (217) 545-1903
Percentage of IMGs in the program: 90%
Minimum USMLE Step 1 Score Requirement: 205
Minimum USMLE Step 2 Score Requirement: 205
Attempts on any step: Must pass on first attempt including CS exam
CS required at time of application: No
USCE Requirement: None
Cut-Off time since graduation: 5 years
Program offers couple match: No
Visas Sponsored or accepted: J1 visa

Loyola University Neurology Residency Program

Specialty: Neurology
Program name: Loyola University Program
Program code: 180-16-21-036

NRMP Code: 1170180C0
Program type: University-based
State: Illinois
Address: Loyola University Medical Center
2160 S First Ave, Maywood, IL 60153
Phone: (708) 216-2687
Fax: (708) 216-5617
Percentage of IMGs in the program: 0%
Minimum USMLE Step 1 Score Requirement: No limits set
Minimum USMLE Step 2 Score Requirement: No limits set
Attempts on any step: No limits set
CS required at time of application: Yes including ECFMG certificate
USCE Requirement: None
Cut-Off time since graduation: 3 years
Program offers couple match: Yes
Visas Sponsored or accepted: J1 visa

University of Illinois College of Medicine at Chicago Neurology Residency Program

Specialty: Neurology
Program name: University of Illinois College of Medicine at Chicago Program
Program code: 180-16-21-035
State: Illinois

Address: University of Illinois Medical Center
912 S Wood St, Chicago, IL 60612-7330
Phone: (312) 996-6906
Fax: (312) 996-4169
Percentage of IMGs in the program: 30%
Minimum USMLE Step 1 Score Requirement: 205
Minimum USMLE Step 2 Score Requirement: 205
Attempts on any step: Must pass on maximum the 2nd attempt including CS exam
CS required at time of application: Yes including ECFMG certificate
USCE Requirement: None
Cut-Off time since graduation: No limits set
Program offers couple match: Yes
Visas Sponsored or accepted: J1 visa

University of Chicago Neurology Residency Neurology Program

Specialty: Neurology
Program name: University of Chicago Program
Program code: 180-16-21-034
NRMP Code: 1160180A0
Program type: University-based
State: Illinois

Address: University of Chicago Hospitals
    5841 S Maryland Ave, Chicago, IL 60637-1470
Phone: (773) 702-0151
Fax: (773) 834-3662
Percentage of IMGs in the program: 40%
Minimum USMLE Step 1 Score Requirement: No limits set (they claim they have it secret)
Minimum USMLE Step 2 Score Requirement: No limits set (they claim they have it secret)
Attempts on any step: No limits set
CS required at time of application: No
USCE Requirement: None
Cut-Off time since graduation: 5 years
Program offers couple match: Yes
Visas Sponsored or accepted: J1 visa and H1 visa

McGaw Medical Center of Northwestern University Neurology Residency Program

Specialty: Neurology
Program name: McGaw Medical Center of Northwestern University Program
Program code: 180-16-21-032
State: Illinois
Address: McGaw Medical Center Northwestern University
    710 N Lake Shore Dr, Chicago, IL

60611
Phone: 312-503-3936
Fax: (312) 908-5073
Percentage of IMGs in the program: 5% (variable)
Minimum USMLE Step 1 Score Requirement: 205
Minimum USMLE Step 2 Score Requirement: 205
Attempts on any step: No limits set
CS required at time of application: No
USCE Requirement: Yes, 1 year
Cut-Off time since graduation: No limits set
Program offers couple match: Yes
Visas Sponsored or accepted: J1 visa and H1b visa

Rush University Medical Center Neurology Residency Program

Specialty: Neurology
Program name: Rush University Medical Center Program
Program code: 180-16-11-033
State: Illinois
Address: Rush University Medical Center
1725 W Harrison St, Chicago, IL 60612
Phone: (312) 942-4500
Fax: (312) 942-2380
Percentage of IMGs in the program: 0%

Minimum USMLE Step 1 Score Requirement: No limits set
Minimum USMLE Step 2 Score Requirement: No limits set
Attempts on any step: No limits set
CS required at time of application: Yes including ECFMG certificate
USCE Requirement: None
Cut-Off time since graduation: 2 years unless clinically active
Program offers couple match: Yes
Visas Sponsored or accepted: J1 visa and H1b visa

Indiana

Indiana University School of Medicine Neurology Residency Program

Specialty: Neurology
Program name: Indiana University School of Medicine Program
Program code: 180-17-21-038

Program type: University-based
State: Indiana
Address: Indiana University School of Medicine
355 W 16th St, Indianapolis, IN 46202
Phone: (317) 963-7408
Fax: (317) 963-7533
Percentage of IMGs in the program: 0%
Minimum USMLE Step 1 Score Requirement: No limits set
Minimum USMLE Step 2 Score Requirement: No limits set
Attempts on any step: No limits set
CS required at time of application: No
USCE Requirement: Yes, at least 1 US LOR
Cut-Off time since graduation: No limits set
Program offers couple match: Yes
Visas Sponsored or accepted: J1 visa

Iowa

University of Iowa Hospitals and Clinics Neurology Residency Program

Specialty: Neurology

Program name: University of Iowa Hospitals and Clinics Program
Program code: 180-18-21-039
State: Iowa
Address: University of Iowa Hospitals and Clinics
200 Hawkins Dr, Iowa City, IA 52242
Phone: (319) 356-8752
Fax: (319) 384-7199
Percentage of IMGs in the program: 30%
Minimum USMLE Step 1 Score Requirement: No limits set
Minimum USMLE Step 2 Score Requirement: No limits set
Attempts on any step: Must pass on maximum 2nd attempt including CS exam
CS required at time of application: Yes including ECFMG certificate
USCE Requirement: Yes including US LOR from neurologist
Cut-Off time since graduation: 4 years
Program offers couple match: Yes
Visas Sponsored or accepted: J1 visa

Kansas

University of Kansas School of Medicine Neurology Residency Program

Specialty: Neurology
Program name: University of Kansas School of Medicine Program
Program code: 180-19-22-040
State: Kansas
Address: University of Kansas Medical Center 3599 Rainbow Blvd, Kansas City, KS 66160-8500
Phone: (913) 588-6970
Fax: (913) 588-6965
Percentage of IMGs in the program: 0% (Occasional one)
Minimum USMLE Step 1 Score Requirement: No limits set
Minimum USMLE Step 2 Score Requirement: No limits set
Attempts on any step: Must pass on the 1st attempt
CS required at time of application: Yes including ECFMG certificate
USCE Requirement: None
Cut-Off time since graduation: 5 years
Program offers couple match: Yes
Visas Sponsored or accepted: J1 visa

Kentucky

University of Louisville Neurology Residency Program

Specialty: Neurology
Program name: University of Louisville Program
Program code: 180-20-21-042
NRMP Code: 1217180A0
Program type: Community-based university affiliated hospital
State: Kentucky
Address: University of Louisville
    500 S Preston St, Louisville, KY 40292-0001
Phone: (502) 852-6328
Fax: (502) 852-6344
Percentage of IMGs in the program: 80%
Minimum USMLE Step 1 Score Requirement: No limits set
Minimum USMLE Step 2 Score Requirement: No limits set
Attempts on any step: No limits set
CS required at time of application: No
USCE Requirement: None
Cut-Off time since graduation: No limits set
Program offers couple match: Yes
Visas Sponsored or accepted: J1 visa

University of Kentucky College of Medicine Neurology Residency Program

Specialty: Neurology
Program name: University of Kentucky College of Medicine Program
Program code: 180-20-21-041
State: Kentucky
Address: University of Kentucky College of Medicine
 740 S Limestone Rd, Lexington, KY 40536
Phone: (859) 218-5038
Fax: (859) 323-5943
Percentage of IMGs in the program: 70%
Minimum USMLE Step 1 Score Requirement: No limits set
Minimum USMLE Step 2 Score Requirement: No limits set
Attempts on any step: No limits set
CS required at time of application: Yes including ECFMG certificate
USCE Requirement: None
Cut-Off time since graduation: No limits set
Program offers couple match: Yes
Visas Sponsored or accepted: J1 visa

Louisiana

Louisiana State University (Shreveport) Neurology Residency Program

Specialty: Neurology
Program name: Louisiana State University (Shreveport) Program
Program code: 180-21-31-153
State: Louisiana
Address: LSU Health Science Center Shreveport
1501 Kings Hwy, Shreveport, LA 71130
Phone: (318) 813-1480
Fax: (318) 675-7805
Percentage of IMGs in the program: 100%
Minimum USMLE Step 1 Score Requirement: No limits set
Minimum USMLE Step 2 Score Requirement: No limits set
Attempts on any step: Must pass maximum on 2nd attempt
CS required at time of application: Yes including ECFMG certificate

USCE Requirement: Yes (Research doesn't count, must be observership in a residency program)
Cut-Off time since graduation: No limits set
Program offers couple match: Yes
Visas Sponsored or accepted: J1 visa

Tulane University Neurology Residency Program

Specialty: Neurology
Program name: Tulane University Program
Program code: 180-21-21-044
NRMP Code: 3073180C0
Program type: University-based
State: Louisiana
Address: Tulane University School of Medicine 1430 Tulane Ave, New Orleans, LA 70112
Phone: (504) 988-2241
Fax: (504) 988-9197
Percentage of IMGs in the program: 30%
Minimum USMLE Step 1 Score Requirement: 235
Minimum USMLE Step 2 Score Requirement: 235
Attempts on any step: Must pass on first attempt including CS exam
CS required at time of application: Yes

USCE Requirement: Yes, 12 months including 3 Neurology rotations and at least 1 Neurology US LOR
Cut-Off time since graduation: 5 years
Program offers couple match: Yes
Visas Sponsored or accepted: No visa

Louisiana State University Neurology Residency Program

Specialty: Neurology
Program name: Louisiana State University Program
Program code: 180-21-21-043
State: Louisiana
Address: LSU Health Science Center New Orleans
1542 Tulane Ave, New Orleans, LA 70112
Phone: (504) 568-4081
Fax: (504) 568-7130
Percentage of IMGs in the program: 50%
Minimum USMLE Step 1 Score Requirement: No limits set
Minimum USMLE Step 2 Score Requirement: No limits set
Attempts on any step: No limits set
CS required at time of application: No
USCE Requirement: None
Cut-Off time since graduation: No limits set

Program offers couple match: No
Visas Sponsored or accepted: J1 visa

Ochsner Clinic Foundation Neurology Residency Program

Specialty: Neurology
Program name: Ochsner Clinic Foundation Program
Program code: 180-21-00-154
Program type: Community-based
State: Louisiana
Address: Ochsner Clinic Foundation
1514 Jefferson Hwy, New Orleans, LA 70121
Phone: (504) 842-7965
Fax: (504) 842-0542
Percentage of IMGs in the program: 50%
Minimum USMLE Step 1 Score Requirement: 200
Minimum USMLE Step 2 Score Requirement: 210
Attempts on any step: Must pass maximum on 2nd attempt including CS exam
CS required at time of application: Yes including ECFMG certificate
USCE Requirement: Yes 1 month
Cut-Off time since graduation: 3 years
Program offers couple match: Yes
Visas Sponsored or accepted: J1 visa

Maryland

University of Maryland Neurology Residency Program

Specialty: Neurology
Program name: University of Maryland Program
Program code: 180-23-31-046
State: Maryland
Address: University of Maryland Medical System
110 S Paca St, Baltimore, MD 21201
Phone: (410) 328-5841
Fax: (410) 328-6651
Percentage of IMGs in the program: 30%
Minimum USMLE Step 1 Score Requirement: No limits set but prefer above 200
Minimum USMLE Step 2 Score Requirement: No limits set
Attempts on any step: No limits set
CS required at time of application: Yes including ECFMG certificate
USCE Requirement: None but preferred
Cut-Off time since graduation: No limits set
Program offers couple match: Yes

Visas Sponsored or accepted: J1 visa

Johns Hopkins University Neurology Residency Program

Specialty: Neurology
Program name: Johns Hopkins University Program
Program code: 180-23-21-045
State: Maryland
Address: Johns Hopkins Hospital
601 N Caroline St, Baltimore, MD 21287-0877
Phone: (410) 502-0817
Fax: (410) 614-1302
Percentage of IMGs in the program: 0%
Minimum USMLE Step 1 Score Requirement: No limits set
Minimum USMLE Step 2 Score Requirement: No limits set
Attempts on any step: No limits set
CS required at time of application: Yes
USCE Requirement: None
Cut-Off time since graduation: No limits set
Program offers couple match: Yes
Visas Sponsored or accepted: J1 visa (H1b visa only for US graduates if they are Foreigners)

Massachusetts

Massachusetts General Hospital/Brigham and Women's Hospital/Harvard Medical School Neurology Residency Program

Specialty: Neurology
Program name: Massachusetts General Hospital/Brigham and Women's Hospital/Harvard Medical School Program
Program code: 180-24-31-050
State: Massachusetts
Address: Massachusetts General Hospital
55 Fruit St, Boston, MA 02114
Phone: (617) 726-1067
Fax: (617) 726-2353
Percentage of IMGs in the program: 10%
Minimum USMLE Step 1 Score Requirement: No limits set
Minimum USMLE Step 2 Score Requirement: No limits set
Attempts on any step: Must pass on first attempt
CS required at time of application: No
USCE Requirement: None
Cut-Off time since graduation: 5 years
Program offers couple match: Yes

Visas Sponsored or accepted: J1 visa and H1b visa

Boston Medical Center Neurology Residency Program

Specialty: Neurology
Program name: Boston Medical Center Program
Program code: 180-24-21-145
State: Massachusetts
Address: Boston University Medical Center
72 E Concord St, Boston, MA 02118-2394
Phone: (617) 638-5309
Fax: (617) 638-5354
Percentage of IMGs in the program: 20%
Minimum USMLE Step 1 Score Requirement: No limits set
Minimum USMLE Step 2 Score Requirement: No limits set
Attempts on any step: No limits set
CS required at time of application: Yes including ECFMG certificate
USCE Requirement: None
Cut-Off time since graduation: No limits set
Program offers couple match: No
Visas Sponsored or accepted: J1 visa

University of Massachusetts Neurology Residency Program

Specialty: Neurology
Program name: University of Massachusetts Program
Program code: 180-24-21-121
NRMP Code: 3050180A0
Program type: University-based
State: Massachusetts
Address: University of Massachusetts Medical School
55 Lake Ave N, Worcester, MA 01655-0318
Phone: (508) 856-3083
Fax: (508) 856-3180
Percentage of IMGs in the program: 40%
Minimum USMLE Step 1 Score Requirement: No limits set
Minimum USMLE Step 2 Score Requirement: No limits set
Attempts on any step: Must pass on first attempt including CS exam
CS required at time of application: Yes
USCE Requirement: Yes
Cut-Off time since graduation: 5 years
Program offers couple match: Yes
Visas Sponsored or accepted: J1 visa

Tufts Medical Center Neurology Residency Program

Specialty: Neurology
Program name: Tufts Medical Center Program
Program code: 180-24-21-051
State: Massachusetts
Address: Tufts Medical Center
800 Washington St, Boston, MA 02111
Phone: (617) 636-2605
Fax: (617) 636-8199
Percentage of IMGs in the program: 35%
Minimum USMLE Step 1 Score Requirement: No limits set
Minimum USMLE Step 2 Score Requirement: No limits set
Attempts on any step: No limits set
CS required at time of application: No
USCE Requirement: None
Cut-Off time since graduation: No limits set
Program offers couple match: Yes
Visas Sponsored or accepted: J1 visa and H1b visa

Beth Israel Deaconess Medical Center/Harvard Medical School Neurology Residency Program

Specialty: Neurology
Program name: Beth Israel Deaconess Medical Center/Harvard Medical School Program
Program code: 180-24-21-049
State: Massachusetts
Address: Beth Israel Deaconess Medical Center
330 Brookline Ave, Boston, MA 02215
Phone: (617) 667-2268
Fax: (617) 667-2987
Percentage of IMGs in the program: 30%
Minimum USMLE Step 1 Score Requirement: No limits set
Minimum USMLE Step 2 Score Requirement: No limits set
Attempts on any step: No limits set
CS required at time of application: Yes including ECFMG certificate
USCE Requirement: Yes
Cut-Off time since graduation: No limits set
Program offers couple match: Yes
Visas Sponsored or accepted: J1 visa

Michigan

Detroit Medical Center/Wayne State University Neurology Residency Program

Specialty: Neurology
Program name: Detroit Medical Center/Wayne State University Program
Program code: 180-25-31-054
State: Michigan
Address: Wayne State University/Detroit Medical Center
 4201 St Antoine Blvd, Detroit, MI 48201
Phone: (313) 745-1302
Fax: (313) 577-4641
Percentage of IMGs in the program: 70%
Minimum USMLE Step 1 Score Requirement: 220
Minimum USMLE Step 2 Score Requirement: 220
Attempts on any step: Must pass on the 1st attempt
CS required at time of application: Yes including ECFMG certificate
USCE Requirement: None
Cut-Off time since graduation: 5 years
Program offers couple match: Yes
Visas Sponsored or accepted: J1 visa

University of Michigan Neurology Residency Program

Specialty: Neurology
Program name: University of Michigan Program
Program code: 180-25-31-052
NRMP Code: 1293180C0
Program type: University-based
State: Michigan
Address: University of Michigan Hospitals and Health Centers
1500 E Medical Center Dr, Ann Arbor, MI 48109-5316
Phone: (734) 936-9556
Fax: (734) 232-6133
Percentage of IMGs in the program: 0%
Minimum USMLE Step 1 Score Requirement: No limits set
Minimum USMLE Step 2 Score Requirement: No limits set
Attempts on any step: No limits set
CS required at time of application: Yes
USCE Requirement: Yes
Cut-Off time since graduation: No limits set
Program offers couple match: Yes
Visas Sponsored or accepted: J1 visa

Sparrow Hospital/Michigan State University Neurology Residency Program

Specialty: Neurology
Program name: Sparrow Hospital/Michigan State University Program
Program code: 180-25-21-149
State: Michigan
Address: Michigan State University
804 Service Rd, East Lansing, MI 48824
Phone: (517) 432-9277
Fax: (517) 432-9414
Percentage of IMGs in the program: 40%
Minimum USMLE Step 1 Score Requirement: No limits set
Minimum USMLE Step 2 Score Requirement: No limits set
Attempts on any step: No limits set
CS required at time of application: Yes including ECFMG certificate
USCE Requirement: Yes 6 months (research counts)
Cut-Off time since graduation: 3 years
Program offers couple match: Yes
Visas Sponsored or accepted: J1 visa

Henry Ford Hospital/Wayne State University Neurology Residency Program

Specialty: Neurology
Program name: Henry Ford Hospital/Wayne State University Program
Program code: 180-25-21-129
NRMP Code: 1300180A0
Program type: Community-based university affiliated hospital
State: Michigan
Address: Henry Ford Hospital
2799 W Grand Blvd, Detroit, MI 48202
Phone: (313) 916-7205
Fax: (313) 916-5117
Percentage of IMGs in the program: 50%
Minimum USMLE Step 1 Score Requirement: No limits set
Minimum USMLE Step 2 Score Requirement: No limits set
Attempts on any step: No limits set
CS required at time of application: Yes including ECFMG certificate
USCE Requirement: None
Cut-Off time since graduation: 3 years
Program offers couple match: Yes
Visas Sponsored or accepted: J1 visa

Grand Rapids Medical Education Partners Neurology Residency Program

Specialty: Neurology
Program name: Grand Rapids Medical Education Partners Program
Program code: 180-25-00-150
NRMP Code: 2077180C0
Program type: Community-based
State: Michigan
Address: Grand Rapids Med Education Partners 25 Michigan Ave NE, Grand Rapids, MI 49503
Phone: (616) 391-3245
Fax: (616) 391-3130
Percentage of IMGs in the program: 40%
Minimum USMLE Step 1 Score Requirement: 215
Minimum USMLE Step 2 Score Requirement: 215
Attempts on any step: Must pass on first attempt
CS required at time of application: No
USCE Requirement: Yes
Cut-Off time since graduation: 5 years
Program offers couple match: Yes
Visas Sponsored or accepted: J1 visa

Minnesota

Mayo Clinic College of Medicine (Rochester) Neurology Residency Program

Specialty: Neurology
Program name: Mayo Clinic College of Medicine (Rochester) Program
Program code: 180-26-21-057
NRMP Code: 1328180C0, 1328180A0
Program type: University-based
State: Minnesota
Address: Mayo Clinic
200 First St SW, Rochester, MN 55905
Phone: (507) 284-4205
Fax: (507) 266-0178
Percentage of IMGs in the program: 0%
Minimum USMLE Step 1 Score Requirement: No limits set
Minimum USMLE Step 2 Score Requirement: No limits set
Attempts on any step: No limits set
CS required at time of application: No
USCE Requirement: None
Cut-Off time since graduation: No limits set
Program offers couple match: Yes
Visas Sponsored or accepted: J1 visa and H1b visa

University of Minnesota Neurology Residency Program

Specialty: Neurology
Program name: University of Minnesota Program
Program code: 180-26-21-055
NRMP Code: 1334180C0
Program type: University-based
State: Minnesota
Address: University of Minnesota Medical Center
420 Delaware St SE, Minneapolis, MN 55455
Phone: (612) 626-6519
Fax: (612) 624-0687
Percentage of IMGs in the program: 50%
Minimum USMLE Step 1 Score Requirement: 210
Minimum USMLE Step 2 Score Requirement: 210
Attempts on any step: No limits set
CS required at time of application: Yes including ECFMG certificate
USCE Requirement: Yes
Cut-Off time since graduation: No limits set
Program offers couple match: Yes
Visas Sponsored or accepted: J1 visa

Mississippi

University of Mississippi Medical Center Neurology Residency Program

Specialty: Neurology
Program name: University of Mississippi Medical Center Program
Program code: 180-27-21-058
NRMP Code: 1957180C0
Program type: University-based
State: Mississippi
Address: University of Mississippi Medical Center
2500 N State St, Jackson, MS 39216
Phone: (601) 984-5514 (601) 984-5500
Fax: (601) 984-5503
Percentage of IMGs in the program: 70%
Minimum USMLE Step 1 Score Requirement: No limits set
Minimum USMLE Step 2 Score Requirement: No limits set
Attempts on any step: No limits set
CS required at time of application: Yes including ECFMG certificate
USCE Requirement: Yes, 1 month observership or rotation in Neurology
Cut-Off time since graduation: No limits set
Program offers couple match: Yes

Visas Sponsored or accepted: J1 visa

Missouri

Washington University/B-JH/SLCH Consortium Neurology Residency Program

Specialty: Neurology
Program name: Washington University/B-JH/SLCH Consortium Program
Program code: 180-28-21-061
State: Missouri
Address: Washington University/Barnes-Jewish Hospital
 660 S Euclid Ave, St Louis, MO 63110
Phone: (314) 362-3296
Fax: (314) 362-9462
Percentage of IMGs in the program: 0% (Occasionally one)
Minimum USMLE Step 1 Score Requirement: No limits set
Minimum USMLE Step 2 Score Requirement: No limits set
Attempts on any step: Must pass on first attempt including CS exam

CS required at time of application: Yes including ECFMG certificate
USCE Requirement: Yes 1 month
Cut-Off time since graduation: 10 years
Program offers couple match: Yes
Visas Sponsored or accepted: J1 visa

St Louis University School of Medicine Neurology Residency Program

Specialty: Neurology
Program name: St Louis University School of Medicine Program
Program code: 180-28-21-060
NRMP Code: 1365180C0
Program type: University-based
State: Missouri
Address: St Louis University School of Medicine 1438 S Grand Blvd, St Louis, MO 63104
Phone: (314) 977-4828
Fax: (314) 977-4877
Percentage of IMGs in the program: 70%
Minimum USMLE Step 1 Score Requirement: 215
Minimum USMLE Step 2 Score Requirement: 215
Attempts on any step: Must pass maximum on 2nd attempt including CS exam

CS required at time of application: Yes including ECFMG certificate
USCE Requirement: None
Cut-Off time since graduation: 8 years
Program offers couple match: Yes
Visas Sponsored or accepted: J1 visa

University of Missouri-Columbia Neurology Residency Program

Specialty: Neurology
Program name: University of Missouri-Columbia Program
Program code: 180-28-21-059
State: Missouri
Address: University of Missouri Hospitals and Clinics
          5 Hospital Dr, Columbia, MO 65212
Phone: (573) 882-2260
Fax: (573) 884-4249
Percentage of IMGs in the program: 90%
Minimum USMLE Step 1 Score Requirement: 215
Minimum USMLE Step 2 Score Requirement: 215
Attempts on any step: Must pass maximum on the 3rd attempt including CS exam
CS required at time of application: No
USCE Requirement: Yes unless graduated within the last 2 years

Cut-Off time since graduation: 5 years unless in residency or clinically active
Program offers couple match: Yes
Visas Sponsored or accepted: J1 visa

Nebraska

University of Nebraska Medical Center College of Medicine/Creighton University Neurology Residency Program

Specialty: Neurology
Program name: University of Nebraska Medical Center College of Medicine/Creighton University Program
Program code: 180-30-21-062
State: Nebraska
Address: University of Nebraska Medical Center 988435 Nebraska Medical Center, Omaha, NE 68198-8435
Phone: (402) 559-5804
Fax: (402) 559-9355
Percentage of IMGs in the program: 100%

Minimum USMLE Step 1 Score Requirement: No limits set
Minimum USMLE Step 2 Score Requirement: No limits set
Attempts on any step: No limits set
CS required at time of application: Yes
USCE Requirement: None
Cut-Off time since graduation: No limits set
Program offers couple match: Yes
Visas Sponsored or accepted: J1 visa and H1b visa

New Hampshire

Dartmouth-Hitchcock Medical Center Neurology Residency Program

Specialty: Neurology
Program name: Dartmouth-Hitchcock Medical Center Program
Program code: 180-32-21-063
NRMP Code: 1377180C0, 1377180A0
Program type: University-based
State: New Hampshire

Address: Dartmouth-Hitchcock Medical Center
One Medical Center Dr, Lebanon, NH 03756
Phone: (603) 650-5458
Fax: (603) 650-6233
Percentage of IMGs in the program: 50%
Minimum USMLE Step 1 Score Requirement: No limits set
Minimum USMLE Step 2 Score Requirement: No limits set
Attempts on any step: No limits set
CS required at time of application: Yes including ECFMG certificate
USCE Requirement: Yes 1 year
Cut-Off time since graduation: No limits set
Program offers couple match: Yes
Visas Sponsored or accepted: J1 visa (and H1b visa for foreign AMGs)

New Jersey

Cooper Medical School of Rowan University/Cooper University Hospital Neurology Residency Program

Specialty: Neurology

Program name: Cooper Medical School of Rowan University/Cooper University Hospital Program
Program code: 180-33-13-158
NRMP Code: 1380180A0
Program type: University-based
State: New Jersey
Address: Cooper Hospital-University Medical Center, Suite 142 E&R Building,
    401 Haddon Ave, Camden, NJ 08103
Phone: (856) 757-7818
Fax: (856) 757-7839
Percentage of IMGs in the program: 40%
Minimum USMLE Step 1 Score Requirement: No limits set
Minimum USMLE Step 2 Score Requirement: No limits set
Attempts on any step: No limits set
CS required at time of application: Yes including ECFMG certificate
USCE Requirement: None
Cut-Off time since graduation: No limits set
Program offers couple match: No
Visas Sponsored or accepted: J1 visa

Rutgers New Jersey Medical School Neurology Residency Program

Specialty: Neurology

Program name: Rutgers New Jersey Medical School Program
Program code: 180-33-21-064
State: New Jersey
Address: Rutgers New Jersey Medical School, 185 S Orange Ave, Newark, NJ 07103-2714
Phone: (973) 972-5209
Fax: (973) 972-5059
Percentage of IMGs in the program: 100%
Minimum USMLE Step 1 Score Requirement: No limits set
Minimum USMLE Step 2 Score Requirement: No limits set
Attempts on any step: No limits set
CS required at time of application: Yes including ECFMG certificate
USCE Requirement: None
Cut-Off time since graduation: No limits set but prefer less than 3 years
Program offers couple match: Yes
Visas Sponsored or accepted: J1 visa

Seton Hall University School of Health and Medical Sciences Neurology Residency Program

Specialty: Neurology
Program name: Seton Hall University School of Health and Medical Sciences Program

Program code: 180-33-21-142
State: New Jersey
Address: NJ NeuroScience Institute JFK Medical Center,
        65 James St, Edison, NJ 08818
Phone: (732) 632-1685
Fax: (732) 632-1584
Percentage of IMGs in the program: 30%
Minimum USMLE Step 1 Score Requirement: 210
Minimum USMLE Step 2 Score Requirement: 210
Attempts on any step: No limits set
CS required at time of application: No
USCE Requirement: None
Cut-Off time since graduation: No limits set
Program offers couple match: No
Visas Sponsored or accepted: J1 visa and H1b visa

Rutgers Robert Wood Johnson Medical School Neurology Residency Program

Specialty: Neurology
Program name: Rutgers Robert Wood Johnson Medical School Program
Program code: 180-33-21-157
NRMP Code: 2918180A0
Program type: University-based

State: New Jersey
Address: Rutgers Robert Wood Johnson Medical School,
125 Paterson St, New Brunswick, NJ 08901
Phone: (732) 235-6017
Fax: (732) 235-7041
Percentage of IMGs in the program: 50%
Minimum USMLE Step 1 Score Requirement: No limits set
Minimum USMLE Step 2 Score Requirement: No limits set
Attempts on any step: No limits set
CS required at time of application: No
USCE Requirement: None
Cut-Off time since graduation: No limits set
Program offers couple match: Yes
Visas Sponsored or accepted: J1 visa

New Mexico

University of New Mexico Neurology Residency Program

Specialty: Neurology

Program name: University of New Mexico Program
Program code: 180-34-21-065
NRMP Code: 1962180A0
Program type: University-based
State: New Mexico
Address: University of New Mexico Health Science Center,
    1 Univ of New Mexico, Albuquerque, NM 87131-0001
Phone: (505) 272-8960
Fax: (505) 272-6692
Percentage of IMGs in the program: 60%
Minimum USMLE Step 1 Score Requirement: 210
Minimum USMLE Step 2 Score Requirement: 210
Attempts on any step: No limits set
CS required at time of application: Yes including ECFMG certificate
USCE Requirement: Yes, 1 year
Cut-Off time since graduation: 5 years
Program offers couple match: Yes

New York

Icahn School of Medicine at Mount Sinai (Beth Israel) Neurology Residency Program

Specialty: Neurology
Program name: Icahn School of Medicine at Mount Sinai (Beth Israel) Program
Program code: 180-35-13-155
NRMP Code: 1470180A0
Program type: University-based
State: New York
Address: Beth Israel Medical Center
10 Union Sq E, New York, NY 10003
Phone: (212) 844-6897
Fax: (212) 844-8407
Percentage of IMGs in the program: 60%
Minimum USMLE Step 1 Score Requirement: No limits set
Minimum USMLE Step 2 Score Requirement: No limits set
Attempts on any step: Must pass on the first attempt
CS required at time of application: No
USCE Requirement: Yes, 1 month
Cut-Off time since graduation: 5 years
Program offers couple match: Yes
Visas Sponsored or accepted: J1 visa (and H1b visa case-to-case)

Albany Medical Center Neurology Residency Program

Specialty: Neurology
Program name: Albany Medical Center Program
Program code: 180-35-21-066
NRMP Code: 1414180C0
Program type: University-based
State: New York
Address: Albany Medical Center
47 New Scotland Ave, Albany, NY 12208
Phone: (518) 262-6488
Fax: (518) 262-6178
Percentage of IMGs in the program: 50%
Minimum USMLE Step 1 Score Requirement: 220
Minimum USMLE Step 2 Score Requirement: 220
Attempts on any step: Must pass on first attempt
CS required at time of application: Yes including ECFMG certificate
USCE Requirement: None
Cut-Off time since graduation: 4 years unless was in residency, research or has experience
Program offers couple match: Yes
Visas Sponsored or accepted: J1 visa

University at Buffalo Neurology Residency Program

Specialty: Neurology
Program name: University at Buffalo Program
Program code: 180-35-21-067
NRMP Code: 3099180C0
Program type: Community-based University affiliated hospital
State: New York
Address: Jacobs Neurological Institute
    100 High St, Buffalo, NY 14203
Phone: (716) 859-3496
Fax: (716) 859-7833
Percentage of IMGs in the program: 80%
Minimum USMLE Step 1 Score Requirement: 210
Minimum USMLE Step 2 Score Requirement: 210
Attempts on any step: No limits set
CS required at time of application: Yes including ECFMG certificate
USCE Requirement: None
Cut-Off time since graduation: No limits set
Program offers couple match: Yes
Visas Sponsored or accepted: J1 visa

Albert Einstein College of Medicine Neurology Residency Program

Specialty: Neurology
Program name: Albert Einstein College of Medicine Program
Program code: 180-35-21-070
NRMP Code: 3153180A0
Program type: University-based
State: New York
Address: Albert Einstein College of Medicine
1410 Pelham Pkwy S, Bronx, NY 10461
Phone: (718) 430-3166
Fax: (718) 430-3237
Percentage of IMGs in the program: 20%
Minimum USMLE Step 1 Score Requirement: 215
Minimum USMLE Step 2 Score Requirement: 215
Attempts on any step: Must pass on first attempt
CS required at time of application: Yes including ECFMG certificate
USCE Requirement: Yes
Cut-Off time since graduation: 6 years
Program offers couple match: Yes
Visas Sponsored or accepted: J1 visa and H1b visa

New York Presbyterian Hospital (Cornell Campus) Neurology Residency Program

Specialty: Neurology
Program name: New York Presbyterian Hospital (Cornell Campus) Program
Program code: 180-35-21-072
State: New York
Address: New York Presbyterian Hospital-Cornell
  525 E 68th St, New York, NY 10065
Phone: (212) 746-6515
Fax: (212) 746-3645
Percentage of IMGs in the program: 30%
Minimum USMLE Step 1 Score Requirement: 210
Minimum USMLE Step 2 Score Requirement: 210
Attempts on any step: No limits set
CS required at time of application: No
USCE Requirement: None
Cut-Off time since graduation: 10 years
Program offers couple match: No
Visas Sponsored or accepted: J1 visa

NSLIJHS/Hofstra North Shore-LIJ School of Medicine Neurology Residency Program

Specialty: Neurology
Program name: NSLIJHS/Hofstra North Shore-LIJ School of Medicine Program
Program code: 180-35-21-074
NRMP Code: 1700180A0
Program type: University-based
State: New York
Address: North Shore University Hospital
300 Community Dr, Manhasset, NY 11030
Phone: (516) 562-2303
Fax: (516) 365-8128
Percentage of IMGs in the program: 50%
Minimum USMLE Step 1 Score Requirement: No limits set
Minimum USMLE Step 2 Score Requirement: No limits set
Attempts on any step: No limits set
CS required at time of application: Yes including ECFMG certificate
USCE Requirement: None
Cut-Off time since graduation: No limits set
Program offers couple match: Yes
Visas Sponsored or accepted: J1 visa and H1b visa

Icahn School of Medicine at Mount Sinai Neurology Residency Program

Specialty: Neurology
Program name: Icahn School of Medicine at Mount Sinai Program
Program code: 180-35-21-075
State: New York
Address: Mount Sinai Medical Centre
One Gustave L Levy Pl, New York, NY 10029
Phone: (212) 241-7074
Fax: (212) 987-7635
Percentage of IMGs in the program: 30%
Minimum USMLE Step 1 Score Requirement: No limits set
Minimum USMLE Step 2 Score Requirement: No limits set
Attempts on any step: Must pass on first attempt
CS required at time of application: Yes including ECFMG certificate
USCE Requirement: Yes with at least 1 US LOR
Cut-Off time since graduation: No limits set
Program offers couple match: Yes
Visas Sponsored or accepted: J1 visa and H1b visa

New York Medical College at Westchester Medical Center Neurology Program

Specialty: Neurology
Program name: New York Medical College at Westchester Medical Center Program
Program code: 180-35-21-076
NRMP Code: 2998180A0
Program type: University-based
State: New York
Address: NYMC Westchester Medical Center Munger Pavilion 4th Floor Room 431, Valhalla, NY 10595
Phone: (914) 594-4293
Fax: (914) 594-4295
Percentage of IMGs in the program: 80%
Minimum USMLE Step 1 Score Requirement: 210
Minimum USMLE Step 2 Score Requirement: 210
Attempts on any step: Must pass maximum on the 2nd attempt
CS required at time of application: Yes including ECFMG certificate
USCE Requirement: Yes
Cut-Off time since graduation: 5 years
Program offers couple match: Yes
Visas Sponsored or accepted: J1 visa and H1b visa

New York University School of Medicine Neurology Residency Program

Specialty: Neurology
Program name: New York University School of Medicine Program
Program code: 180-35-21-077
NRMP Code: 2978140P1
Program type: University-based
State: New York
Address: New York University Medical Center
240 E 38th St, New York, NY 10016
Phone: (212) 263-8223
Fax: (646) 501-9248
Percentage of IMGs in the program: 10% (Varies)
Minimum USMLE Step 1 Score Requirement: 200
Minimum USMLE Step 2 Score Requirement: No limits set
Attempts on any step: No limits set
CS required at time of application: No
USCE Requirement: None
Cut-Off time since graduation: No limits set
Program offers couple match: Yes
Visas Sponsored or accepted: J1 visa and H1b visa

SUNY Health Science Center at Brooklyn Neurology Residency Program

Specialty: Neurology
Program name: SUNY Health Science Center at Brooklyn Program
Program code: 180-35-21-079
State: New York
Address: SUNY Downstate Medical Center
450 Clarkson Ave, Brooklyn, NY 11203-2098
Phone: (718) 270-4232
Fax: (718) 270-3840
Percentage of IMGs in the program: 50%
Minimum USMLE Step 1 Score Requirement: 220
Minimum USMLE Step 2 Score Requirement: 220
Attempts on any step: Must pass on first attempt
CS required at time of application: Yes including ECFMG certificate
USCE Requirement: Yes
Cut-Off time since graduation: 10 years
Program offers couple match: Yes
Visas Sponsored or accepted: J1 visa

SUNY at Stony Brook Neurology Residency Program

Specialty: Neurology
Program name: SUNY at Stony Brook Program
Program code: 180-35-21-081
NRMP Code: 2919180A0
Program type: University-based
State: New York
Address: SUNY Stony Brook University
101 Nicolls Road, Stony Brook, NY 11794-8121
Phone: (631) 444-7878
Fax: (631) 706-4484
Percentage of IMGs in the program: 80%
Minimum USMLE Step 1 Score Requirement: No limits set
Minimum USMLE Step 2 Score Requirement: No limits set
Attempts on any step: Must pass maximum on 2nd attempt but no failures accepted for CS
CS required at time of application: No
USCE Requirement: None
Cut-Off time since graduation: No limits set but must be clinically active within the last 5 years
Program offers couple match: Yes
Visas Sponsored or accepted: J1 visa

SUNY Upstate Medical University Neurology Residency Program

Specialty: Neurology
Program name: SUNY Upstate Medical University Program
Program code: 180-35-21-083
State: New York
Address: SUNY Upstate Medical University
750 E Adams St, Syracuse, NY 13210
Phone: (315) 464-5357
Fax: (315) 464-5355
Percentage of IMGs in the program: 90%
Minimum USMLE Step 1 Score Requirement: 220
Minimum USMLE Step 2 Score Requirement: 220
Attempts on any step: Must pass from the first attempt
CS required at time of application: Yes including ECFMG certificate
USCE Requirement: None but preferred
Cut-Off time since graduation: 5 years preferred
Program offers couple match: Yes
Visas Sponsored or accepted: J1 visa

New York Presbyterian Hospital (Columbia Campus) Neurology Residency Program

Specialty: Neurology
Program name: New York Presbyterian Hospital (Columbia Campus) Program
Program code: 180-35-31-071
State: New York
Address: New York Presbyterian Hospital-Columbia
        710 W 168th St, New York, NY 10032
Phone: (212) 305-1338
Fax: (212) 305-6978
Percentage of IMGs in the program: 10% (Variable)
Minimum USMLE Step 1 Score Requirement: 230
Minimum USMLE Step 2 Score Requirement: 230
Attempts on any step: No limits set
CS required at time of application: Yes including ECFMG certificate
USCE Requirement: None
Cut-Off time since graduation: No limits set
Program offers couple match: Yes
Visas Sponsored or accepted: J1 visa

University of Rochester Neurology Residency Program

Specialty: Neurology
Program name: University of Rochester Program
Program code: 180-35-31-082
State: New York
Address: University of Rochester Medical Center
 601 Elmwood Ave, Rochester, NY 14642
Phone: (585) 275-2545
Fax: (585) 244-2529
Percentage of IMGs in the program: 15% (Varies)
Minimum USMLE Step 1 Score Requirement: 200
Minimum USMLE Step 2 Score Requirement: 205
Attempts on any step: Must pass on the first attempt
CS required at time of application: No
USCE Requirement: None
Cut-Off time since graduation: Within the last 16 months at time of application
Program offers couple match: Yes
Visas Sponsored or accepted: J1 visa

North Carolina

Wake Forest University School of Medicine Neurology Residency Program

Specialty: Neurology
Program name: Wake Forest University School of Medicine Program
Program code: 180-36-21-086
State: North Carolina
Address: Wake Forest Baptist Medical Center
Medical Center Blvd, Winston-Salem, NC 27157
Phone: (336) 716-2317
Fax: (336) 716-7790
Percentage of IMGs in the program: 0%
Minimum USMLE Step 1 Score Requirement: No limits set
Minimum USMLE Step 2 Score Requirement: No limits set
Attempts on any step: No limits set
CS required at time of application: Yes including ECFMG certificate
USCE Requirement: Yes, 1 year
Cut-Off time since graduation: No limits set
Program offers couple match: Yes
Visas Sponsored or accepted: J1 visa

Duke University Hospital Neurology Residency Program

Specialty: Neurology
Program name: Duke University Hospital Program
Program code: 180-36-21-085
State: North Carolina
Address: Duke University Medical Center
Bryan Research Center
311 Research Drive, Durham, NC 27710
Phone: (919) 684-5870
Fax: (919) 684-0131
Percentage of IMGs in the program: 20%
Minimum USMLE Step 1 Score Requirement: No limits set
Minimum USMLE Step 2 Score Requirement: No limits set
Attempts on any step: No limits set
CS required at time of application: Yes including ECFMG certificate
USCE Requirement: None
Cut-Off time since graduation: No limits set
Program offers couple match: Yes
Visas Sponsored or accepted: No visa

University of North Carolina Hospitals Neurology Residency Program

Specialty: Neurology
Program name: University of North Carolina Hospitals Program
Program code: 180-36-11-084
State: North Carolina
Address: University of North Carolina Hospitals 170 Manning Dr, Chapel Hill, NC 27599-7025
Phone: (919) 966-8162
Fax: (919) 966-2922
Percentage of IMGs in the program: 10%
Minimum USMLE Step 1 Score Requirement: No limits set
Minimum USMLE Step 2 Score Requirement: No limits set
Attempts on any step: No limits set
CS required at time of application: No
USCE Requirement: None
Cut-Off time since graduation: No limits set
Program offers couple match: Yes
Visas Sponsored or accepted: J1 visa

Ohio

Wright State University Boonshoft School of Medicine Neurology Residency Program

Specialty: Neurology
Program name: Wright State University Boonshoft School of Medicine Program
Program code: 180-38-00-144
State: Ohio
Address: Miami Valley Hospital
128 E Apple St, Dayton, OH 45409
Phone: (937) 208-3424
Fax: (937) 208-3413
Percentage of IMGs in the program: 0%
Minimum USMLE Step 1 Score Requirement: 210
Minimum USMLE Step 2 Score Requirement: 210
Attempts on any step: Must pass on first attempt
CS required at time of application: Yes including ECFMG certificate
USCE Requirement: None
Cut-Off time since graduation: 5 years
Program offers couple match: Yes
Visas Sponsored or accepted: No visa

Cleveland Clinic Foundation Neurology Residency Program

Specialty: Neurology
Program name: Cleveland Clinic Foundation Program
Program code: 180-38-11-090
NRMP Code: 1968180C0
Program type: University-based
State: Ohio
Address: Cleveland Clinic
9500 Euclid Ave, Cleveland, OH 44195-5242
Phone: (216) 444-2945
Fax: (216) 445-9908
Percentage of IMGs in the program: 50%
Minimum USMLE Step 1 Score Requirement: 210
Minimum USMLE Step 2 Score Requirement: 210
Attempts on any step: No limits set
CS required at time of application: Yes including ECFMG certificate
USCE Requirement: Yes, 1 month
Cut-Off time since graduation: No limits set
Program offers couple match: Yes
Visas Sponsored or accepted: J1 visa and H1b visa

University of Cincinnati Medical Center/College of Medicine Neurology Rresidency Program

Specialty: Neurology
Program name: University of Cincinnati Medical Center/College of Medicine Program
Program code: 180-38-21-088
NRMP Code: 1548180C0
Program type: University-based
State: Ohio
Address: University Hospital University of Cincinnati
  260 Stetson St, Cincinnati, OH 45267-0525
Phone: (513) 558-2968
Fax: (513) 558-4887
Percentage of IMGs in the program: 30%
Minimum USMLE Step 1 Score Requirement: No limits set
Minimum USMLE Step 2 Score Requirement: No limits set
Attempts on any step: No limits set
CS required at time of application: Yes including ECFMG certificate
USCE Requirement: None
Cut-Off time since graduation: No limits set
Program offers couple match: Yes
Visas Sponsored or accepted: J1 visa

Case Western Reserve University/University Hospitals Case Medical Center Neurology Residency Program

Specialty: Neurology
Program name: Case Western Reserve University/University Hospitals Case Medical Center Program
Program code: 180-38-21-089
NRMP Code: 1552180C0
Program type: University-based
State: Ohio
Address: University Hospitals Case Medical Center
   11100 Euclid Ave, Cleveland, OH 44106
Phone: (216) 844-5550
Fax: (216) 983-0792
Percentage of IMGs in the program: 70%
Minimum USMLE Step 1 Score Requirement: 210
Minimum USMLE Step 2 Score Requirement: 210
Attempts on any step: Must pass on first attempt
CS required at time of application: Yes including ECFMG certificate
USCE Requirement: None
Cut-Off time since graduation: 5 years

Program offers couple match: Yes
Visas Sponsored or accepted: J1 visa

Ohio State University Hospital Neurology Residency Program

Specialty: Neurology
Program name: Ohio State University Hospital Program
Program code: 180-38-21-092
NRMP Code: 1566180C0
Program type: University-based
State: Ohio
Address: Ohio State University Wexner Medical Center
     395 W 12th Ave, Columbus, OH 43210-1250
Phone: (614) 293-6872
Fax: (614) 293-4688
Percentage of IMGs in the program: 20%
Minimum USMLE Step 1 Score Requirement: 230
Minimum USMLE Step 2 Score Requirement: 230
Attempts on any step: No limits set
CS required at time of application: Yes including ECFMG certificate
USCE Requirement: Yes, 1 month
Cut-Off time since graduation: 5 years
Program offers couple match: Yes

Visas Sponsored or accepted: J1 visa

University of Toledo Neurology Residency Program

Specialty: Neurology
Program name: University of Toledo Program
Program code: 180-38-21-143
NRMP Code: 1579180C0
Program type: University-based
State: Ohio
Address: University of Toledo Medical Center
3000 Arlington Ave, Toledo, OH 43614
Phone: (419) 383-3661
Fax: (419) 383-3093
Percentage of IMGs in the program: 100%
Minimum USMLE Step 1 Score Requirement: 210
Minimum USMLE Step 2 Score Requirement: 210
Attempts on any step: No limits set
CS required at time of application: Yes including ECFMG certificate
USCE Requirement: Yes, 1 month
Cut-Off time since graduation: 5 years
Program offers couple match: Yes
Visas Sponsored or accepted: J1 visa

Oklahoma

University of Oklahoma Health Sciences Center Neurology Residency Program

Specialty: Neurology
Program name: University of Oklahoma Health Sciences Center Program
Program code: 180-39-21-141
NRMP Code: 1588180C0
Program type: University-based
State: Oklahoma
Address: University of Oklahoma Health Sciences Center
　　　　920 Stanton L Young Blvd, Oklahoma City, OK 73104
Phone: (405) 271-4113
Fax: (405) 271-5723
Percentage of IMGs in the program: 40%
Minimum USMLE Step 1 Score Requirement: 218
Minimum USMLE Step 2 Score Requirement: 218
Attempts on any step: No limits set
CS required at time of application: Yes including ECFMG certificate
USCE Requirement: None

Cut-Off time since graduation: No limits set, but no more than 5 years since the last clinical activity
Program offers couple match: Yes
Visas Sponsored or accepted: J1 visa

Oregon

Oregon Health & Science University Neurology Residency Program

Specialty: Neurology
Program name: Oregon Health & Science University Program
Program code: 180-40-31-095
NRMP Code: 1599180A0
Program type: University-based
State: Oregon
Address: Oregon Health & Science University 3181 SW Sam Jackson Park Rd, Portland, OR 97239-3098
Phone: (503) 494-5753
Fax: (503) 418-8373
Percentage of IMGs in the program: 20%

Minimum USMLE Step 1 Score Requirement: No limits set
Minimum USMLE Step 2 Score Requirement: No limits set
Attempts on any step: Prefer no failures
CS required at time of application: Yes including ECFMG certificate
USCE Requirement: Yes, 1 month
Cut-Off time since graduation: 5 years
Program offers couple match: Yes
Visas Sponsored or accepted: J1 visa and H1b visa

Pennsylvania

Geisinger Health System Neurology Residency Program

Specialty: Neurology
Program name: Geisinger Health System Program
Program code: 180-41-00-166
State: Pennsylvania
Address: Geisinger Medical Center
100 N Academy Ave, Danville, PA 17822-1403

Phone: (570) 214-9175
Fax: (570) 214-9175
Percentage of IMGs in the program: 20%
Minimum USMLE Step 1 Score Requirement: No limits set
Minimum USMLE Step 2 Score Requirement: No limits set
Attempts on any step: No limits set
CS required at time of application: No
USCE Requirement: None
Cut-Off time since graduation: No limits set
Program offers couple match: Yes
Visas Sponsored or accepted: J1 visa and H1b visa

Penn State Milton S Hershey Medical Center Neurology Residency Program

Specialty: Neurology
Program name: Penn State Milton S Hershey Medical Center Program
Program code: 180-41-11-096
State: Pennsylvania
Address: Penn State Milton S Hershey Medical Center
    30 Hope Dr, Hershey, PA 17033-0859
Phone: (717) 531-8692
Fax: (717) 531-0384
Percentage of IMGs in the program: 20%

Minimum USMLE Step 1 Score Requirement: No limits set, above 220 is desirable
Minimum USMLE Step 2 Score Requirement: No limits set, above 220 is desirable
Attempts on any step: No limits set
CS required at time of application: Yes
USCE Requirement: Yes, 1 month within the past 2 years with 1 neurology US LOR
Cut-Off time since graduation: 5 years
Program offers couple match: Yes
Visas Sponsored or accepted: J1 visa

Drexel University College of Medicine/Hahnemann University Hospital Neurology Residency Program

Specialty: Neurology
Program name: Drexel University College of Medicine/Hahnemann University Hospital Program
Program code: 180-41-21-097
NRMP Code: 1849180A0
Program type: University-based
State: Pennsylvania
Address: Hahnemann University Hospital, 245 North 15th Street, MS 423, Philadelphia, PA 19102-1192
Phone: (215) 762-4592
Fax: (215) 762-3161

Percentage of IMGs in the program: 80%
Minimum USMLE Step 1 Score Requirement: No limits set
Minimum USMLE Step 2 Score Requirement: No limits set
Attempts on any step: No limits set
CS required at time of application: Yes including ECFMG certificate
USCE Requirement: None but previous Internal medicine residency for IMGs encouraged
Cut-Off time since graduation: 5 years
Program offers couple match: Yes
Visas Sponsored or accepted: J1 visa

Temple University Hospital Neurology Residency Program

Specialty: Neurology
Program name: Temple University Hospital Program
Program code: 180-41-21-100
NRMP Code: 1646180C0
Program type: University-based
State: Pennsylvania
Address: Temple University Hospital
3401 N Broad St, Philadelphia, PA 19140
Phone: (215) 707-3094
Fax: (215) 707-3831
Percentage of IMGs in the program: 70%

Minimum USMLE Step 1 Score Requirement:
No limits set but above 220 is desirable
Minimum USMLE Step 2 Score Requirement:
No limits set but above 220 is desirable
Attempts on any step: No limits set
CS required at time of application: Yes including ECFMG certificate
USCE Requirement: None
Cut-Off time since graduation: No limits set
Program offers couple match: Yes
Visas Sponsored or accepted: J1 visa and H1b visa

Thomas Jefferson University Neurology Residency Program

Specialty: Neurology
Program name: Thomas Jefferson University Program
Program code: 180-41-21-101
State: Pennsylvania
Address: Thomas Jefferson University Hospital, 901 Walnut St, Philadelphia, PA 19107
Phone: (215) 955-9425
Fax: (215) 503-4347
Percentage of IMGs in the program: 20%
Minimum USMLE Step 1 Score Requirement: No limits set

Minimum USMLE Step 2 Score Requirement: No limits set
Attempts on any step: Must pass on first attempt
CS required at time of application: Yes including ECFMG certificate
USCE Requirement: None
Cut-Off time since graduation: 5 years
Program offers couple match: Yes
Visas Sponsored or accepted: J1 visa and H1b visa

University of Pennsylvania Neurology Residency Program

Specialty: Neurology
Program name: University of Pennsylvania Program
Program code: 180-41-21-102
Program type: University-based
State: Pennsylvania
Address: Hospital of University of Pennsylvania
3400 Spruce St, Philadelphia, PA 19104
Phone: (215) 662-3370
Fax: (215) 662-3362
Percentage of IMGs in the program: 0%
Minimum USMLE Step 1 Score Requirement: 210

Minimum USMLE Step 2 Score Requirement: 210
Attempts on any step: Must pass on first attempt
CS required at time of application: Yes including ECFMG certificate
USCE Requirement: Yes, 1 month within the past 6 months
Cut-Off time since graduation: 2 years
Program offers couple match: Yes
Visas Sponsored or accepted: J1 visa

UPMC Medical Education Neurology Residency Program

Specialty: Neurology
Program name: UPMC Medical Education Program
Program code: 180-41-21-103
State: Pennsylvania
Address: University of Pittsburgh Medical Center
    3471 Fifth Ave, Pittsburgh, PA 15213
Phone: (412) 648-2022
Fax: (412) 624-2302
Percentage of IMGs in the program: 0% (occasionally one)
Minimum USMLE Step 1 Score Requirement: No limits set

Minimum USMLE Step 2 Score Requirement: No limits set
Attempts on any step: Must pass on first attempt
CS required at time of application: No
USCE Requirement: None
Cut-Off time since graduation: No limits set
Program offers couple match: Yes
Visas Sponsored or accepted: J1 visa and H1b visa

Allegheny General Hospital-Western Pennsylvania Hospital Medical Education Consortium (AGH) Neurology Residency Program

Specialty: Neurology
Program name: Allegheny General Hospital-Western Pennsylvania Hospital Medical Education Consortium (AGH) Program
Program code: 180-41-21-140
 State: Pennsylvania
Address: Allegheny General Hospital,
            490 E North Ave, Pittsburgh, PA 15212-9986
Phone: (412) 359-6527
Fax: (412) 359-8477
Percentage of IMGs in the program: 30%

Minimum USMLE Step 1 Score Requirement: 210
Minimum USMLE Step 2 Score Requirement: 210
Attempts on any step: No limits set
CS required at time of application: No
USCE Requirement: Yes, 1 month
Cut-Off time since graduation: 10 years
Program offers couple match: Yes
Visas Sponsored or accepted: J1 visa

Albert Einstein Healthcare Network Neurology Residency Program

Specialty: Neurology
Program name: Albert Einstein Healthcare Network Program
Program code: 180-41-33-162
NRMP Code: 1631180A0
Program type: Community-based University affiliated hospital
State: Pennsylvania
Address: Albert Einstein Medical Center
　　　　　5501 Old York Rd, Philadelphia, PA 19141
Phone: (215) 456-4961
Fax: (215) 456-0386
Percentage of IMGs in the program: 80%
Minimum USMLE Step 1 Score Requirement: No limits set

Minimum USMLE Step 2 Score Requirement: No limits set
Attempts on any step: Must pass on first attempt
CS required at time of application: No
USCE Requirement: None
Cut-Off time since graduation: No limits set
Program offers couple match: Yes
Visas Sponsored or accepted: J1 visa and H1b visa

Rhode Island

Brown University Neurology Residency Program

Specialty: Neurology
Program name: Brown University Program
Program code: 180-43-21-131
NRMP Code: 1677180A0
Program type: University-based
State: Rhode Island
Address: Rhode Island Hospital
110 Lockwood St, Providence, RI 02903

Phone: (401) 444-4364
Fax: (401) 444-8781
Percentage of IMGs in the program: 0%
Minimum USMLE Step 1 Score Requirement: No limits set
Minimum USMLE Step 2 Score Requirement: No limits set
Attempts on any step: No limits set
CS required at time of application: Yes
USCE Requirement: None
Cut-Off time since graduation: No limits set
Program offers couple match: Yes
Visas Sponsored or accepted: J1 visa

South Carolina

Palmetto Health/University of South Carolina School of Medicine Neurology Residency Program

Specialty: Neurology
Program name: Palmetto Health/University of South Carolina School of Medicine Program
Program code: 180-45-12-164
NRMP Code: 1681180C0

Program type: Community-based University affiliated hospital
State: South Carolina
Address: University of South Carolina School of Medicine
8 Medical Park, Columbia, SC 29203
Phone: (803) 545-6072
Fax: (803) 545-5061
Percentage of IMGs in the program: 40%
Minimum USMLE Step 1 Score Requirement: No limits set
Minimum USMLE Step 2 Score Requirement: No limits set
Attempts on any step: No limits set
CS required at time of application: Yes including ECFMG certificate
USCE Requirement: None
Cut-Off time since graduation: No limits set
Program offers couple match: Yes
Visas Sponsored or accepted: No visa

Medical University of South Carolina Neurology Residency Program

Specialty: Neurology
Program name: Medical University of South Carolina Program
Program code: 180-45-21-105
State: South Carolina

Address: Medical University of South Carolina
96 Jonathan Lucas St, Charleston, SC 29425-2232
Phone: (843) 792-3222
Fax: (843) 792-8626
Percentage of IMGs in the program: 25%
Minimum USMLE Step 1 Score Requirement: 220
Minimum USMLE Step 2 Score Requirement: 220
Attempts on any step: Must pass maximum on the 2nd attempt
CS required at time of application: No
USCE Requirement: Yes
Cut-Off time since graduation: No limits set
Program offers couple match: Yes
Visas Sponsored or accepted: J1 visa

Tennessee

University of Tennessee Neurology Residency Program

Specialty: Neurology
Program name: University of Tennessee Program
Program code: 180-47-21-106

NRMP Code: 1844180A0
Program type: University-based
State: Tennessee
Address: University of Tennessee Health Science Center,
   Department of Neurology Room 415,
   855 Monroe Ave, Memphis, TN 38163
Phone: (901) 448-6661
Fax: (901) 448-7440
Percentage of IMGs in the program: 50%
Minimum USMLE Step 1 Score Requirement: 230
Minimum USMLE Step 2 Score Requirement: 230
Attempts on any step: Must pass on first attempt including CS exam
CS required at time of application: No
USCE Requirement: Yes but not a strict requirement
Cut-Off time since graduation: 3 years, unless clinically active then 5 years.
Program offers couple match: Yes
Visas Sponsored or accepted: J1 visa

Vanderbilt University Neurology Residency Program

Specialty: Neurology

Program name: Vanderbilt University Program
Program code: 180-47-21-107
NRMP Code: 1702180C0
Program type: University-based
State: Tennessee
Address: Vanderbilt University Medical Center,
Suite A-0118 Med Center North,
1161 21st Ave S, Nashville, TN 37232
Phone: (615) 936-1567
Fax: (615) 936-2675
Percentage of IMGs in the program: 5%
Minimum USMLE Step 1 Score Requirement: 220
Minimum USMLE Step 2 Score Requirement: 220
Attempts on any step: No limits set
CS required at time of application: Yes including ECFMG certificate
USCE Requirement: Yes including 2 US LORs
Cut-Off time since graduation: No limits set
Program offers couple match: Yes
Visas Sponsored or accepted: J1 visa and H1b visa

Texas

Scott and White Memorial Hospital Neurology Residency Program

Specialty: Neurology
Program name: Scott and White Memorial Hospital Program
Program code: 180-48-00-167
State: Texas
Address: Scott and White Memorial Hospital
2401 S 31st St, Temple, TX 76508
Phone: (254) 724-4179
Fax: (254) 724-5692
Percentage of IMGs in the program: 0%
Minimum USMLE Step 1 Score Requirement: No limits set
Minimum USMLE Step 2 Score Requirement: No limits set
Attempts on any step: No limits set
CS required at time of application: Yes including ECFMG certificate
USCE Requirement: None
Cut-Off time since graduation: No limits set
Program offers couple match: Yes
Visas Sponsored or accepted: J1 visa

University of Texas Medical Branch Hospitals Neurology Residency Program

Specialty: Neurology
Program name: University of Texas Medical Branch Hospitals Program
Program code: 180-48-11-109
NRMP Code: 1714180A0
Program type: University-based
State: Texas
Address: University of Texas Medical Branch Hospitals
   301 University Blvd, Galveston, TX 77555-0539
Phone: (409) 772-8031
Fax: (409) 772-6940
Percentage of IMGs in the program: 70%
Minimum USMLE Step 1 Score Requirement: No limits set
Minimum USMLE Step 2 Score Requirement: No limits set
Attempts on any step: No limits set
CS required at time of application: No
USCE Requirement: None
Cut-Off time since graduation: No limits set
Program offers couple match: Yes
Visas Sponsored or accepted: J1 visa and H1b visa

University of Texas Southwestern Medical School (Austin) Neurology Residency Program

Specialty: Neurology
Program name: University of Texas Southwestern Medical School (Austin) Program
Program code: 180-48-12-156
Program type: Community-based University affiliated hospital
State: Texas
Address: Seton Brain and Spine Institute
　　　　　1400 North IH-35, Austin, TX 78701
Phone: (512) 324-7890
Fax: (512) 324-8212
Percentage of IMGs in the program: 25%
Minimum USMLE Step 1 Score Requirement: 225
Minimum USMLE Step 2 Score Requirement: 225
Attempts on any step: Must pass maximum on the 2nd attempt
CS required at time of application: No
USCE Requirement: Yes, 1 month preferred
Cut-Off time since graduation: 5 years
Program offers couple match: Yes
Visas Sponsored or accepted: J1 visa

Methodist Hospital (Houston) Neurology Residency Program

Specialty: Neurology
Program name: Methodist Hospital (Houston) Program

Program code: 180-48-12-160
State: Texas
Address: Methodist Neurological Institute
6560 Fannin St, Houston, TX 77030
Phone: (713) 441-3336
Fax: (713) 790-5079
Percentage of IMGs in the program: 60%
Minimum USMLE Step 1 Score Requirement: 230
Minimum USMLE Step 2 Score Requirement: 230
Attempts on any step: Must pass on first attempt
CS required at time of application: Yes including ECFMG certificate
USCE Requirement: None
Cut-Off time since graduation: 5 years
Program offers couple match: Yes
Visas Sponsored or accepted: No visa

Texas Tech University (Lubbock) Neurology Residency Program

Specialty: Neurology
Program name: Texas Tech University (Lubbock) Program
Program code: 180-48-13-163
NRMP Code: 2973180C0
Program type: University-based
State: Texas

Address: Texas Tech University HSC Lubbock
3601 4th St, Lubbock, TX 79430
Phone: (806) 743-3832
Fax: (806) 743-2974
Percentage of IMGs in the program: 80%
Minimum USMLE Step 1 Score Requirement: No limits set
Minimum USMLE Step 2 Score Requirement: No limits set
Attempts on any step: No limits set
CS required at time of application: Yes including ECFMG certificate
USCE Requirement: Yes
Cut-Off time since graduation: No limits set
Program offers couple match: Yes
Visas Sponsored or accepted: J1 visa

University of Texas Southwestern Medical School Neurology Residency Program

Specialty: Neurology
Program name: University of Texas Southwestern Medical School Program
Program code: 180-48-21-108
State: Texas
Address: University of Texas Southwestern Medical Center
5323 Harry Hines Blvd, Dallas, TX 75390-9036

Phone: (214) 648-4775
Fax: (214) 648-5080
Percentage of IMGs in the program: 20% (variable)
Minimum USMLE Step 1 Score Requirement: No limits set
Minimum USMLE Step 2 Score Requirement: No limits set
Attempts on any step: No limits set
CS required at time of application: Yes including ECFMG certificate
USCE Requirement: Yes, 1 month
Cut-Off time since graduation: 5 years
Program offers couple match: Yes
Visas Sponsored or accepted: J1 visa

Baylor College of Medicine Neurology Residency Program

Specialty: Neurology
Program name: Baylor College of Medicine Program
Program code: 180-48-21-110
NRMP Code: 1716180C0
Program type: University-based
State: Texas
Address: Baylor College of Medicine
6501 Fannin St, Houston, TX 77030-3498
Phone: (713) 798-6151

Fax: (713) 798-8530
Percentage of IMGs in the program: 10%
Minimum USMLE Step 1 Score Requirement: No limits set
Minimum USMLE Step 2 Score Requirement: No limits set
Attempts on any step: Must pass on the first attempt
CS required at time of application: Yes including ECFMG certificate
USCE Requirement: None
Cut-Off time since graduation: No limits set
Program offers couple match: Yes
Visas Sponsored or accepted: J1 visa

University of Texas Health Science Center at San Antonio Neurology Residency Program

Specialty: Neurology
Program name: University of Texas Health Science Center at San Antonio Program
Program code: 180-48-21-112
NRMP Code: 1722180A0
Program type: University-based
State: Texas
Address: University of Texas HSC San Antonio 8300 Floyd Curl Dr, San Antonio, TX 78229
Phone: (210) 567-1324

Fax: (210) 567-4659
Percentage of IMGs in the program: 70%
Minimum USMLE Step 1 Score Requirement: No limits set
Minimum USMLE Step 2 Score Requirement: No limits set
Attempts on any step: No limits set
CS required at time of application: Yes including ECFMG certificate
USCE Requirement: Yes, 1 month
Cut-Off time since graduation: No limits set
Program offers couple match: Yes
Visas Sponsored or accepted: J1 visa

University of Texas at Houston Neurology Residency Program

Specialty: Neurology
Program name: University of Texas at Houston Program
Program code: 180-48-31-111
NRMP Code: 2923180C0
Program type: University-based
State: Texas
Address: University of Texas Medical School Houston
    6431 Fannin St, Houston, TX 77030
Phone: (713) 500-7052
Percentage of IMGs in the program: 50%

Minimum USMLE Step 1 Score Requirement: 225
Minimum USMLE Step 2 Score Requirement: 225
Attempts on any step: No limits set
CS required at time of application: Yes including ECFMG certificate
USCE Requirement: None
Cut-Off time since graduation: No limits set
Program offers couple match: Yes
Visas Sponsored or accepted: J1 visa

Utah

University of Utah Neurology Residency Program

Specialty: Neurology
Program name: University of Utah Program
Program code: 180-49-21-113
NRMP Code: 1732180C0
Program type: University-based
State: Utah
Address: University of Utah Medical Center, Department of Neurology CNC 175,
 175 N Medical Dr, Salt Lake City, UT 84132-2305
Phone: (801) 585-5405

Fax: (801) 581-4192
Percentage of IMGs in the program: 30%
Minimum USMLE Step 1 Score Requirement: No limits set
Minimum USMLE Step 2 Score Requirement: No limits set
Attempts on any step: No limits set
CS required at time of application: Yes including ECFMG certificate
USCE Requirement: None
Cut-Off time since graduation: No limits set
Program offers couple match: Yes
Visas Sponsored or accepted: J1 visa

Vermont

University of Vermont/Fletcher Allen Health Care Neurology Residency Program

Specialty: Neurology
Program name: University of Vermont/Fletcher Allen Health Care Program
Program code: 180-50-11-114
NRMP Code:
Program type:
State: Vermont

Address: University of Vermont FAHC, Department of Neurology,
89 Beaumont Ave, Burlington, VT 05405
Phone: (802) 656-4588
Fax: (802) 656-5678
Percentage of IMGs in the program: 60%
Minimum USMLE Step 1 Score Requirement: No limits set
Minimum USMLE Step 2 Score Requirement: No limits set
Attempts on any step: No limits set
CS required at time of application: Yes including ECFMG certificate
USCE Requirement: Yes at least 1 month within the last 2 years
Cut-Off time since graduation: 2 years
Program offers couple match: Yes
Visas Sponsored or accepted: J1 visa

Virginia

Virginia Commonwealth University Health System Neurology Residency Program

Specialty: Neurology

Program name: Virginia Commonwealth University Health System Program
Program code: 180-51-21-116
Program type: University-based
State: Virginia
Address: VCU Health System, PO Box 980599 Room 6-017,
        1101 E Marshall St, Richmond, VA 23298-0599
Phone: (804) 828-9583
Fax: (804) 828-6373
Percentage of IMGs in the program: 60%
Minimum USMLE Step 1 Score Requirement: No limits set
Minimum USMLE Step 2 Score Requirement: No limits set
Attempts on any step: No limits set
CS required at time of application: Yes including ECFMG certificate
USCE Requirement: Yes at least 3months in the last 4 years
Cut-Off time since graduation: 4 years
Program offers couple match: Yes
Visas Sponsored or accepted: J1 visa

University of Virginia Neurology Residency Program

Specialty: Neurology

Program name: University of Virginia Program
Program code: 180-51-11-115
Program type: University-based
State: Virginia
Address: University of Virginia Health System, Neurology Department,
          PO Box 800394, Charlottesville, VA 22908
Phone: (434) 924-5818
Fax: (434) 982-1726
Percentage of IMGs in the program: 5%
Minimum USMLE Step 1 Score Requirement: No limits set
Minimum USMLE Step 2 Score Requirement: No limits set
Attempts on any step: No limits set
CS required at time of application: No
USCE Requirement: None
Cut-Off time since graduation: No limits set
Program offers couple match: Yes
Visas Sponsored or accepted: J1 visa

Washington

University of Washington Neurology Residency Program

Specialty: Neurology

Program name: University of Washington Program
Program code: 180-54-21-117
NRMP Code: 1918180C0
Program type: University-based
State: Washington
Address: University of Washington School of Medicine, Box 356465,
   1959 NE Pacific St, Seattle, WA 98195
Phone: (206) 685-1281
Fax: (206) 685-8850
Percentage of IMGs in the program: 15%
Minimum USMLE Step 1 Score Requirement: No limits set
Minimum USMLE Step 2 Score Requirement: No limits set
Attempts on any step: Must pass on first attempt
CS required at time of application: Yes including ECFMG certificate
USCE Requirement: Yes at least 1 month within the last 2 years
Cut-Off time since graduation: No limits set
Program offers couple match: Yes
Visas Sponsored or accepted: J1 visa and H1b visa

West Virginia

West Virginia University Neurology Residency Program

Specialty: Neurology
Program name: West Virginia University Program
Program code: 180-55-11-118
NRMP Code: 1837180C0
Program type: University-based
State: West Virginia
Address: West Virginia University HSC, PO Box 9180,
   One Medical Center Dr, Morgantown, WV 26506-9180
Phone: (304) 293-2342
Fax: (304) 293-3352
Percentage of IMGs in the program: 60%
Minimum USMLE Step 1 Score Requirement: No limits set
Minimum USMLE Step 2 Score Requirement: No limits set
Attempts on any step: No limits set
CS required at time of application: No
USCE Requirement: None
Cut-Off time since graduation: 10 years
Program offers couple match: Yes
Visas Sponsored or accepted: J1 visa

Wisconsin

Medical College of Wisconsin Affiliated Hospitals Neurology Residency Program

Specialty: Neurology
Program name: Medical College of Wisconsin Affiliated Hospitals Program
Program code: 180-56-21-120
NRMP Code: 1784180C0
Program type: University-based
State: Wisconsin
Address: Froedtert Memorial Lutheran Hospital, Department of Neurology,
 9200 W Wisconsin Ave, Milwaukee, WI 53226
Phone: (414) 805-5254
Fax: (414) 805-5252
Percentage of IMGs in the program: 50%
Minimum USMLE Step 1 Score Requirement: No limits set
Minimum USMLE Step 2 Score Requirement: No limits set
Attempts on any step: Must pass on first attempt
CS required at time of application: Yes

USCE Requirement: Yes with at least 1 US Neurology LOR
Cut-Off time since graduation: 5 years
Program offers couple match: Yes
Visas Sponsored or accepted: J1 visa and H1b visa

University of Wisconsin Neurology Residency Program

Specialty: Neurology
Program name: University of Wisconsin Program
Program code: 180-56-21-119
NRMP Code: 1779180C0
Program type: University-based
State: Wisconsin
Address: University of Wisconsin Hospital and Clinics, Neurology Program,
　　　1685 Highland Ave, Madison, WI 53705
Phone: (608) 265-4300
Fax: (608) 263-0412
Percentage of IMGs in the program: 40%
Minimum USMLE Step 1 Score Requirement: No limits set
Minimum USMLE Step 2 Score Requirement: No limits set
Attempts on any step: No limits set

CS required at time of application: Yes including ECFMG certificate
USCE Requirement: None
Cut-Off time since graduation: No limits set
Program offers couple match: Yes
Visas Sponsored or accepted: J1 visa

I wish you good luck.

Thank you for buying our book.

Please, Please and Please take a minute to review our book on Amazon.

Match A Doc
Residency Guide

www.matchadoc.com

www.ingramcontent.com/pod-product-compliance
Lightning Source LLC
Chambersburg PA
CBHW051918170526
45168CB00001B/448